BICYCLING THE CONTINENTAL DIVIDE
Slice of Heaven, Taste of Hell

by

Frosty Wooldridge

authorHOUSE®

AuthorHouse™
1663 Liberty Drive, Suite 200
Bloomington, IN 47403
www.authorhouse.com
Phone: 1-800-839-8640

First published by AuthorHouse 8/9/2007

ISBN: 978-1-4343-0457-5 (e)
ISBN: 978-1-4343-0456-8 (sc)

Printed in the United States of America
Bloomington, Indiana

This book is printed on acid-free paper.

Dedicated to:

John Brown

To his passion for life;
For his gift to his students;
For his courage to live;
For the miracle of his spirit.

CONTENTS

After riding two coast-to-coast bicycle tours across America and three other border to border adventures from Canada to Mexico—this ride down the Continental Divide provided the greatest continuous challenge as well as the most profound scenery of all my rides across the United States.

Beginning in Banff International Park, the road provided astounding mountain vistas for 2,500 miles all the way to the Mexican border. In addition to the wilderness, a host of historical figures popped up along the way. We crossed paths with Lewis and Clark, the Blackfeet, Navajo, Geronimo, Jim Bridger, Buffalo Bill, Billy the Kid and many other western legends.

This is not an easy ride as we crossed the Continental Divide nine times. We pressed the pedals hard for many days and many passes. In northwestern Colorado, we skipped over to Utah for a fantastic experience in Arches National Park and Canyonlands. There's nothing quite like Abbey Country and "DESERT SOLITAIRE."

At one point, a tourist asked, "Wouldn't it be easier to ride on flat land?"

"Tell me two things that are exciting about riding across flat country?" Denis asked.

The guy couldn't think of one.

It's true! Give me a mountain to climb on my bike and I'm the happiest rider in the world. I'll take the Andes, Himalaya, Rocky Mountains, Swiss Alps or Pyrenees over flat land.   With great challenges come great rewards. At the same time, a few moments made us question our sanity for riding such a mountainous route. No matter! Pedal forward!

In this adventure, two struggles contended for our emotions. Doctors diagnosed our friend John Brown with cancer two weeks before the ride. John stayed home with chemo and radiation while Denis and I rode the mountain passes with John's battle on our minds. It made for an interesting perspective about those of us living life and others struggling to stay alive.

You may find flashbacks, musings and philosophical questions asked and answered in this book. You may be provoked into questioning life on many levels. Zen and the art of bicycle adventure await.

One aspect soars throughout this adventure. You will discover fun and be inspired to ride it yourself. When you do, the time of your life on your bicycle awaits you!

Frosty Wooldridge
Louisville, Colorado

CHAPTER 1 — GLASSES FOGGED, FINGERS FROZEN,
LEGS SHREDDED--AND WE ARE STILL HAVING FUN?

"When I was young and the urge to be someplace else was upon me, I was assured by mature people that maturity would cure this itch. When years described me as mature; the remedy prescribed was middle age. In middle age, I was assured that greater age would calm my fever and now that I am fifty-eight, perhaps senility will do the job. Nothing has worked. Four hoarse blasts of a ship's whistle still raise the hair on the back of my neck and set my feet to tapping. The sound of a jet, an engine warming up, even the clopping of shod hooves on pavement brings on the ancient shudder, the dry mouth and vacant eye, the hot palms and the churn in the stomach high up under the rib cage. In other words, I don't improve; in further words, once a traveler, always a traveler. I fear the disease is incurable. When the virus of restlessness begins to take possession of a wayward man, and the road away from here seems broad and straight and sweet...he must go."

John Steinbeck

From where we stood astride our bikes, we faced a 4,000-foot climb to the top of 9,400 foot Dunraven Pass. Denis figured three hours. We began in a slight mist which gave way to overcast skies, but no rain. The road led up and up--still further up. We followed the pavement along a stream, through the pine forests and along an aspen grove--still upward toward a battleship gray sky. Cool winds shivered our flesh. The road snaked along the hillsides toward the pass. Stroke after stroke--we climbed. We ate, drank and pressed the pedals. We cranked upward at four miles per hour. We gained altitude from 6,000 to 7,000 to 8,000 feet and beyond.

We labored up the flank of that mountain--with a grass-filled valley on our left. Several backpackers stood with binoculars perched on tripods. One lady said, "That's a grizzly over there next to the woods."

Everyone jerked their eyes to the spot. I strained to see the magnificent beast. Down across the green grasses, over a river and along the woods--a huge, tan-shouldered, anvil-shaped head grizzly bear rummaged in a dead tree stump looking for lunch. Before me, he wrenched his head upward as if toying with some meal he captured. He looked big, maybe 900 pounds of hair, tooth and claw. I watched him for several minutes.

Later, I jumped back astride my bike 'Condor' and continued upward out of the valley and into a burned forest with skeleton trees standing dead by the millions. Their tan trunks, devoid of bark and needles, hung on the landscape like faceless soldiers in a war against a fire they lost. Lost? Not really! A new generation of pines shot from the forest floor in a fresh rekindling of life.

We pedaled through the woods as the road meandered along the side of Washburn Mountain--still moving upward. Darn! Would this climb ever end?

"How far to the pass do you think?" I asked Denis.

"Keep pedaling forever and you will succeed to the top," he replied.

From the backside of forever at 6:30 p.m., we reached the pass with a threatening storm rumbling toward us. Clouds mushroomed in the valley filled with dead trees. A mist soaked the air as if it was a giant steam room at the gym. Darkness crept into the wilds. We stopped to put on our rain gear and gloves. As we jumped on our bikes, rain fell. Big, fat, cruel raindrops hit full force with a cold wind driving them. Down the mountain we rolled. The rain increased as we dropped into deep, green forests along a river. Still further from the 9,400-foot Dunraven Pass, we flew down that valley from our high perch.

"You crazy man," I muttered to myself. "This is miserable. I'm freezing. My glasses are fogged, nearly blinding me, my feet are soaked, my fingers feel like icicles, my butt hurts like my doctor had shot up both my cheeks with penicillin, my legs feel numb, I'm 52 years old, I've got a runny nose, my shoulders ache, and I'm flying down a 9,400-foot mountain on a bicycle in a heavy rainstorm."

Even I had to pause at times wondering why I willingly tortured my body. Was it fun? Like I told that Swiss lady in the camper van days before, "Bicycle adventure is drama. It is the stuff of life. It is struggle, courage, tenacity, victory and fulfillment that make it spiritual, and oh, so marvelous. I love that first bird singing in the morning and the last chirp at night not to mention the coyotes howling their songs."

How could I deny myself these pleasures of the spirit in this overly mechanized world?

Yes, Jack London, I too, am a meteor--blazing happily, white-hot with searing excitement across the sky of my life.

But at that moment, I felt miserable. It sucked!

Shivering like a naked man in a snowstorm, I thought back to how I got myself into that predicament of riding the Continental Divide....

CHAPTER 2 — TOO SILENT TO BE REAL

*"By passionately believing in what
doesn't exist; you create it."*

Ernest Holmes

A certain sadness shrouded my thoughts as our silver-winged aircraft descended through the clouds into Calgary, Canada. Below, green fields sprinkled with cows and horses created a verdant farmland mosaic across the vastness of the conquered wilderness of North America. Wisps of whiteness streaked past my window as I sat contemplating yet another grand adventure on my bicycle.

But this time, my long time friend, John Brown, who had anticipated this journey with great expectations, remained at home in Australia with a bad case of cancer. It tormented my mind for a month--and my concern about his Titanic struggle sobered my thoughts. We remain ephemeral creatures--so vulnerable to the whims of disease, accident and birth. Knowing John as I have for the past 15 years, he would win this battle against cancer. I promised I would ride with him on this great Canada to Mexico journey when he became well again.

He and I had more campfires to share--and that would drive him to the goal of health. I could only imagine his daily struggle with chemotherapy. He battled with his heart and mind; fighting to maintain the living force. For every day that passed, my thoughts and prayers moved toward him.

After the plane touched down, I headed out the gate to meet our mutual and long time friend, Denis LeMay of Quebec, Canada. Denis, a Frenchman, stood waiting for me with a happy grin on his face. We had not seen each other in 12 years. He looked great, but I noticed the years on his face. We were no longer young men--but in the last third of our lives. The wrinkles had set in, as well as adding years to our eyes. Hopefully, wisdom had replaced the speculations of youth.

We caught a shuttle with a young adventurer named Brett. He had traveled to South America, Australia and Europe. He shared many ideas about his life path. "No office cubicle for me," he said. "I've got to be outside."

It's amazing how powerful we are at 27 years. I remember my own brashness at the same age. He will go far beyond those who sit and click their remotes.

Brett took us to a Banff National Park campground on that hot August day where we pitched our tents and crawled into our bags for a good night's sleep. Denis said goodnight in French, and I responded in kind. We had met when I took French studies at Laval University in 1981, but I was still barely an infant when it came to speaking the French language. Denis would have to communicate with me in English. And, as I would find out, he presented some hilarious ways of speaking English.

We woke up to one of those brilliant blue skies dropping down from the heavens to profile gray rock mountains and green forests. All about us, aspen trees fluttered in the morning breeze.

We pulled the bikes out of the boxes and assembled them. First, we locked the wheels into the dropouts. We screwed racks into place along with seats and handlebars. We loaded panniers into place, added safety flags, and filled our water bottles.

Before mounting our touring mountain bikes, we toasted John Brown. We raised our cups to his life.

"A toast to John," Denis said, his hand on a cup of hot chocolate.

"Yes, he will ride with us in spirit," I said, raising my own cup.

Shortly before our journey, John wrote me about going through his retirement physical after teaching for 33 years. After all those decades of education and community involvement, he retired to chase life on his terms. Only life had other things in store for him. The doctors discovered lymphoma cancer in his neck. He underwent immediate surgery to take out the growth.

Thereafter, his doctors prescribed chemotherapy for the next ten weeks. Later, he faced radiation therapy.

We biked across America in 1984. He wanted to ride again, and so, we made plans for the toughest mountainous course in North America--the "Spine of the Rockies." We expected to cross the Continental Divide nine times in 2500 miles. We expected to pedal our iron steeds through six national parks and numerous monuments. This ride offers the best challenges for men and women who love to push the pedals, sweat, ride and eat. The views: breathtaking and priceless!

But he wouldn't be going on it. Not this time, but next time.

We rolled the bikes out of the campground and into the town of Banff. It nestled into the rugged Canadian Rockies. We inflated the bike tires and bought food. The route to Radium Springs on Highway 1 followed a noisy expressway for 20 miles. We rode along a green river with thick forests that crept all the way up to high mountain country. A quiet serendipity of deep, silent green pervaded the landscape.

Each tree shot skyward. In unison, they created a living carpet—moving with the land, rolling up the canyons and growing beyond the hanging valleys. All so quiet yet powerful! Beyond the trees, towering peaks breached the skyline. From there, cliffs dropped out of the mist, and in the distance--deep, dark battleship gray clouds moved through towering rocks, hiding and then exposing pristine granite cathedrals. One looked like the Notre Dame Cathedral--with powerful flanks, flying buttresses and windows exposing the soul of the wilderness.

At Route 93, we turned south. Another dark storm front advanced. Within minutes, hail pelted us and rain fell.

"I thought you promised clear skies and sunshine," Denis blurted to me as he stopped to pull on his rain gear.

"Hey," I said, grinning. "This is your country and you're supposed to have sunshine in August. I was counting on you to provide it. This sucks!"

Denis said, "Don't be sad."

"I'm not," I said, struggling into my rain pants. "It's just a little weather party."

The rain thickened as we mounted our bikes and pedaled up the mountain. Thoreau wrote a piece on the weather: "We are rained and snowed on with gems. What a world we live in! Where are the jewelers' shops? There is nothing more handsome than a raindrop or snowflake or dewdrop. I may say that the maker of the world exhausts his skill with each snowflake and dewdrop he sends down. We think that the one mechanically coheres and that the other simply flows together and falls, but in truth, they are the product of 'enthusiasm', the children of ecstasy, finished with the artist's utmost skill."

We pushed into that storm. As with all inclement weather, we endured it. We didn't curse it, but it didn't thrill us. On a bike, we pedaled at the mercy, or should

I say the acceptance of our natural surroundings. No protection! We equaled the birds, fish, elk, wolves and grizzlies. We rolled through mosquito land! That's one of the things about bicycle touring; you return into nature's arms. That, to me, is a glorious rendition of life. For, how much closer can you rub shoulders with life, than riding daily in the raw power of nature's grasp?

My friend, John Muir strapped himself to a tree once in the middle of a vicious storm in Yosemite. He wanted to 'know' how it felt to be a tree in a storm. It nearly killed him, but he wrote, "But if I should be fated to walk no more with nature, be compelled to leave all I most love in the wilderness, to return to civilization and be twisted into the characterless cable of society--then these sweet, free cumberless rovings will be as chinks and slits on life's horizon, through which I may obtain glimpses of the treasures that lie in the creator's wilds beyond my reach."

Like my friend, I too, wanted to escape my cabled existence in this runaway, high speed society--if only for a short time.

We kept pounding the pedals up a six percent grade where the road, enshrouded in mist, vanished into the rain-covered sky. Gray colored our world. Sweat soaked us. That's one of the conditions with bike touring in the rain. We kept dry from the rain, but we perspired so much we soaked ourselves anyway. Either way, we were wet. After several miles, we reached a high ridge where an abandoned summer camp with cabins nestled into the woods.

"That's enough today," Denis said, motioning to me.

"Let's make this home for tonight," I said. "We'll call it, 'Camp Abandoned Cabins.'"

Denis stopped at an old phone booth that was outside the gates, and made a call.

"What are you calling for?" I asked.

"RV rentals," he said. "I'm not sure I want to ride my bike this whole trip....we need a backup plan."

"I'll kill myself before I travel in a motor home," I said, with a stiff upper lip.

"Bad idea, huh?" Denis said, grinning with his fake phone call.

"Let's get past the gates and get out of sight," I said.

We pitched our tents before cooking dinner. How good can a hot cup of noodle soup taste? Incredibly delicious when you're so hungry you could eat a church banquet table down to the tablecloth--and lick the dishes clean enough to put back into the cupboard! We fired up the one-burner stoves and served ourselves hot chocolate, rice and beans, along with wheat bread, several peanut butter sandwiches and some cookies.

We hung the food bags up in trees off in the woods. No sense giving Mr. Grizzly any excuse to saunter into camp for a late night snack.

Next day, fog rolled in with mist wafting through the trees. We couldn't see through the thick gray low level cloud. We decided to build a fire and cook our oatmeal for breakfast.

We chatted while waiting for our food to cook. We talked about AIDS in Africa, and war in Iraq. We realized how life is random. A person's fate is tied to his/her birth, country, parents, brains, luck and/or bad luck.

We broke camp at mid-morning and headed into the mist. Fog-shrouded trees pointed to a gray sky. Our vision reached 60 yards at most. The mist boiled through the valley as we descended Vermilion Pass at 5480 feet. We coasted down into the fog until we stopped at a big sign for the Continental Divide. While taking some shots, Denis stood with the mist all around when he turned toward the road.

"Yow!" he yelled. "Look at that!"

I turned, "Wow! What a mountain!"

We looked through a sudden window in the clouds to a snow-covered peak one mile over our heads. Gray mist framed it--and the sun shone off its highest peak. I took a shot. Denis raised his camera, but missed a shot as the mist moved in and a gray void once again filled the sky.

We continued down the pass on a three percent grade, which allowed us effortless pedaling. Not far along the way, a turquoise river flowed along the road. On both sides of the highway, clouds broke open, revealing green mantled mountains that led up to gray rock peaks at 12,000 feet. Like the yellow brick road in, "The Wizard of Oz", we enjoyed pink fireweed growing along our route. For miles on either side of the road, deep green flourished as if we were the first explorers into that area. We soon rode out of Banff and into Kootenai National Park. The wilderness grew ever thicker--the quietness more profound.

Gordon Lightfoot wrote about it in a railroad song when he sang, "The deep, dark forests were too silent to be real." For me, this grand display of nature touched my soul--even gave me a glimmer of hope that humanity has enough intelligence to save itself from itself. If we can create national parks, we can create ways to preserve all life on this planet. We pedaled at a good pace with nearly flat to down-hill incline all the way through the morning. We stopped at a lodge where we repaired a slow leak in my back tire.

Denis met a French Canadian couple from Montreal. They chatted for ten minutes.

We rode 25 miles the day before so our legs and butts adapted to the long days of pedaling ahead of us. I found myself thinking about John Brown often and how he would be loving this ride for it was full of grand mountain scenery of gargantuan dimensions. He would have loved to power his bike along those magnificent roads where an elk, deer or moose could pop up at any time. He loved fresh air and the pure joy of pedaling his touring machine.

After cranking the bikes all day along the flower-lined road of fireweed and white and yellow daisies, we climbed up St. Clair Pass and out of Kootenai Valley.

We dripped sweat up a hot, arduous climb until we reached a vista at the top. After pictures, we continued our climb to Olive Lake. Looking back north over the valley, we witnessed nothing but green wilderness that reached to gray peaks. The thickness of the trees masked where we had been. The distance from the peaks that ran from north to south was at least five miles and the peaks themselves were 12,000 feet. It was like we had ridden through a green half-pipe that snow boarders use to do their tricks.

We stopped to camp for the night. Olive Lake turned out to be a spring fed, shallow, crystal clear lake surrounded by ferns, flowers and trees growing down to the shore line. The spring proved a peaceful, bubbling and enchanting spot where Tinker Bell might fly out and touch us with her magic dust. We took baths in the lake and shuddered with the icy cold water. No matter how cold, it felt better to be clean.

We cooked noodle soup. Along with rice and beans, we chowed down on the last of our bread. Even though it was the same food, it tasted better and better. We burned 5,000 calories that day. The usual person burns about 2,200 calories each day. As we sat there on an ancient picnic table, mosquitoes buzzed us, but, because we were too mean and ornery for eating, they flew away for other prey.

We dubbed that area, "Camp Peaceful Easy Feeling."

CHAPTER 3 — NO STATIC STATE
OF PERFECTION POSSIBLE

"The summer--no sweeter was ever;
The sunshiny woods all athrill;
The grayling aleap in the river,
The bighorn asleep on the hill.

The strong life that never knows harness;
The wilds where the caribou call;
The freshness, the freedom, the farness---
O God! How I'm stuck on it all.

It's the great, big, broad land way up yonder,
It's the forests where silence has lease;
It's the beauty that thrills me with wonder;
It's the stillness that fills me with peace."

Robert Service

While riding today, we read why the highway department placed little orange flags along the road where a deer, elk, fox, bird, cougar, bear, mountain sheep, skunk, raccoon or other animal had died from trying to cross the highway. It was a nice gesture, but most people do not slow down for animals. They shrug and call it "road kill."

I've always wondered why we don't fence off highways and provide migration tunnels for animals to cross safely. We do it for human beings. Unfortunately, we don't value our fellow creatures as much as we do ourselves. During the day, I saw hundreds of flags. It looked like a Macy's Thanksgiving Day parade. Flags rippled in the breeze, but in this case, they signaled the death of other living beings unfortunate enough to be going about their own business of living when someone roared along in a two-ton vehicle and snuffed out their lives.

I'm reminded what my friend John Muir wrote about animals, "Of the many advantages of farm life for boys--one of the greatest is the gaining of real knowledge of animals, as fellow mortals, learning to respect them and love them, and even to win some of their love. Thus God-like sympathy grows and thrives, and spreads far beyond the teachings of churches and schools--where too often, the mean, blinding, loveless doctrine is taught that animals have neither mind nor soul, have no rights that we are bound to respect, and were made only for man, to be petted, spoiled, slaughtered, or enslaved."

We saw a buck in the morning, but upon seeing us, he bolted into the woods. He bounded away, moving gracefully, as if blessed with wings for momentary flight--his white tail erect and his body throbbing with life.

John Muir also wrote, "How many hearts with warm blood in them are beating under cover of the woods, and how many teeth and eyes are shining? A multitude of animal people, intimately related to us, but of whose lives we know almost nothing, are as busy about their own affairs as we are about ours."

In the woods, we heard a woodpecker knocking at a tree. A crow called as he flew over our heads. A meadowlark sang her melodious song. A breeze rustled the aspen and made that familiar sound as it rushed through the pines. Somewhere in there, a nasty skunk stunk up the place, but we passed his 'air' space and got on with our normal breathing as quickly as possible.

Thinking back to our camp that morning, I thought that Olive Lake presented us with a paradise of tranquility where little fishes swam in glass clear water, and trees cleaned the air so well we couldn't see it. Back in Denver, you can see the color brown most days across the skyline. But at Olive Lake, the pine scents of the forest delighted my nostrils.

We awakened to crows, sparrows and butterflies. The grass outside our tents glistened with dew while slugs and spiders covered our tents. Thank goodness for enclosed tents. I'd hate to have a slug crawling across my face at night. It would mess up my breathing if it got stuck in my nose!

Back to the moment, my bike coasted quickly downhill toward Radium Hot Springs. We followed a river downward as we threaded the needle through a narrow canyon. The town of Radium featured flowers in front of every building.

The road out of Radium led through a valley fenced by 12,000 foot mountains on the east and west sides. We ran the gauntlet for the entire morning. A bright sun and hot weather caused quite a sweat on our brows. Sweat soaked our shirts.

At mid day, we pedaled past a lake that sourced the headwaters of the mighty Columbia River. It stretched for miles and we pedaled to where it emptied into a stream that would become the most powerful river on the west coast. We enjoyed a brilliant ride along those sparkling waters.

Later, we stopped at a small grocery where we bought some cold juice. Outside, a small, cold pond with a deck offered us a spot to cool our feet off. A bunch of ducks lounged in the water. We took off our shoes and socks.

"Oh man, this is great!" I said.

"Nice way to take heat from our feet," Denis said, sipping on his grapefruit drink.

An older couple sat down to sink their feet into the pool, too. They had cycled half way around the USA that summer from Pennsylvania to Maine, and over to Victoria, Canada. They were heading south toward

Mexico to complete the ride in southern climes. The tall man sported a gray beard while his wife stood lithe and sparkly. I told them about John's cancer. He had been a doctor for 36 years and said chemo was effective in killing half as many patients as it saved. Not exciting news to me! The conversation turned to travel and they headed south to complete a circuit around the USA.

"Retirement," he said, "is everything!"

We pedaled 55 miles to a quiet pond in the woods that featured all the trimmings of a quaint country picture. When we arrived, trees hid it from our sight, but as we followed the dirt road, glass-still waters came into view. Thoreau must have lived there. Reeds grew out from the shore where turtles basked in the sun as they lounged on sun bleached old tree trunks. Yellow flowered lilies covered the water in green patches. Several frogs slept on the bigger lily pads. Dragonflies flew everywhere like confetti in a New York parade. A dozen Mallard ducks paddled their way across the waters where they created open ended triangles with their wakes. Out in the middle, a man in an orange rubber suit floated in a green inner tube while fly-fishing. Where in the heck did he come from? He lofted his line across the water in a rhythmic, poetic motion much like the boys in the movie, "A River Runs Through It." Never was there a more peaceful place under a crimson sky than the scene before us. As the sun set, a crescent moon reflected off the waters.

We enjoyed peace, spirit and solitude. At moments like that, in that magic, everything felt right with the world. It helped me understand where Thoreau gathered his wisdom. Few people live by a pond and think great thoughts like that. Today, there is a highway nearby with trucks roaring past or a plane overhead blasting the silence into submission. If not that, then another human is playing the top 40 hits on his CD. If it's a teenager, they've got rap, acid rock, heavy metal or some other form of ear pain at peak decibels.

I remembered a quote by some brilliant mind, "To many people, the wilderness is little more than a retreat from the tensions of civilization. To others, it is a testing place--a vanishing frontier where man/woman can rediscover basic values. And to a few, the wilderness is nothing less than an almost holy source of self-renewal. But for every man, woman and child, the ultimate lesson is simply this: humanity's fate is inextricably linked to that of the world at large, and to all of the other creatures that live upon it."

We pitched our tents, cooked dinner and fell asleep. What happened to the guy in the orange suit? Heck, he might have drowned for all we knew!

As usual, in the morning, I picked up a sack of litter left by former campers who trashed the place. It made me feel good to leave a place nicer than I found it. Denis acted the same way. We must have picked up more trash in the wilderness than most New York garbage collection crews.

Back on the highway south, we enjoyed a slight tailwind. We passed an electrical transfer station with its wires and conductors.

"Let's turn in there," I said to Denis.

"Why?" he asked.

"I need a charge," I joked.

Just another road joke that died on the vine!

We talked while pedaling.

Denis had traveled through Africa, Russia, India, Europe, Australia, South America and North America. I delighted in his stories.

We followed a line of mountains on our left and a nearly flat road that took a few dives and steep climbs when it hit a river valley. When we coasted down, it took seconds, but when we cranked up a mountain, it sometimes took hours.

We cut from Route 93 onto Route 3 and back to 93 again. We stopped at the Fort Steel Resort and cleaned up in their restroom. A good shave smoothed our faces.

I tried to pump up my tire at the air station, but the thing malfunctioned and I lost air. That forced me to get out my hand pump and do it the old fashioned way. We headed out along a highway lined with trees and farmer's fields full of corn and wheat. We saw big barns, cows and farmers riding their tractors, cutting hay, bailing and loading it onto flatbed wagons.

By lunch time, we stopped at an old grocery store with picnic tables out front. While we sat there, two 14 year old boys shoved a couple of wads of chewing tobacco into their mouths. Normally, I grit my teeth and go about my business, but they were so young, I felt compelled to say something. I walked over and talked to them about the dangers of throat, mouth and stomach cancer from chewing tobacco. I tried to give them some ideas on what happens to thousands of kids who chew so young and how they catch cancer and suffer disfiguring operations in their late 30s and 40s. I talked about how it would cut short their lives when they were having their own kids, and that they would be unable to enjoy their lives when cancer hit. They listened, but I know they didn't hear me.

We pedaled into a hot afternoon with sweat and toil- -rolling our iron steeds toward the US border. About five miles before the border, we stopped at a deserted cabin where we found a spigot and dry ground. Voila! "Camp Peace and Quiet." We pitched our tents and washed in the ice cube temperature water. No matter how cold the water, on a bike trip, I will jump in and freeze to death to become clean. After making myself as miserable as possible, I dry off and feel like a million dollars. It must be some masochistic/sadistic form of self-abuse and ultimate joy when I get clean.

We watched a brilliant sunset with gold-purple clouds overhead and a crescent moon sliding across the sky in slow motion. When the sun dropped below the horizon, mosquitoes attacked from nowhere. I sat with rain gear on and plastic bags over my bare feet. The little demons puncture through Lycra, but they can't bite through nylon and plastic. Ha! There's a T-shirt I bought in the Yukon once that had a big mosquito on the front and read, "Air Show--June through September."

Denis wrote in his own journal about the day's events. It was a quiet time on our bikes--no big deal. We talked about John and his battle...maybe how he was winning it. He must win it so he can go with us on the next bicycle adventure.

The world spins and we move along. Denis and I talked about how fast world events raced and how we must adapt. I try to keep it slow by keeping my life as simple as possible. Yet, computers and high speed everything, along with meetings and schedules, make the clock our god.

I once heard a politician say, "We want things to be the way they used to be."

People long for the good old days. They wax nostalgic. I say, "Don't waste your time." Nothing is ever the same. As Alfred Whitehead wrote, "The foundation of all understanding...is that no static maintenance of perfection is possible. This axiom is rooted in the nature of the universe. Advance or decline is the only choice to mankind. The pure conservative is fighting against the essence of the universe."

Chapter 4 — Claws Four Inches Long

"Bears are made of the same dust as we, and breathe the same winds and drink of the same waters. A bear's days are warmed by the same sun, and his dwellings are over-domed by the same blue sky, and his life turns and ebbs with heart-pulsings like ours, and was poured from the same First Fountain. And, whether he at last goes to our stingy heaven or not, he has terrestrial immortality. His life not long, not short, knows no beginning, no ending. To him life unstinted, unplanned is above the accidents of time and his years, markless and boundless, equal eternity."

John Muir

Denis looked down at his packs while securing them to his bicycle.

"I think they're growing and getting bigger," he said.

Food filled our packs as our appetites grew with more of our energy being expended in the mountains. Cranking a fully loaded mountain bike with water and gear burned a lot of calories. We carried 70 pounds and sometimes more. Denis looked dismayed at his burgeoning panniers.

Denis is funny. His humor is fast and he must use the English language, which makes it harder because he doesn't know the idioms. Nonetheless, he keeps me laughing.

We broke camp and ate at a picnic table. Back on the road, we fell into our rhythm and rolled into the cool morning. In a half-hour, we reached the USA border. "Welcome to Montana," the sign read. A big, puffy Border Patrol officer, twice the size of the usual truck driver, asked us a few questions and waved us on our way.

Route 93 headed straight south with mountains lining both sides of the highway. I dropped down on my aero bars and relaxed in that racing position. It was the first time I had used the elbow bars. They created a very relaxing position and easier on my arms. I could change to four different positions on my handlebars at any time.

We rode through the blistering hot morning until an emerald green lake begged us to jump in with all our clothes on. We did! Nothing like the pure childlike joy of swimming through crystal clear waters. After drying off, we remounted our bikes and headed down the road. The rest of the day gave us a straight shot up and down-hills to White Fish.

Two ladies pedaling north didn't even stop to say "Hi." Nonetheless, it was nice to see women on adventure highway.

We stopped at a grocery. A nice juicy melon tasted great on the steps of the store. It dripped sweet and cold while filling us.

We passed a lot of farms, cows and houses on our way southward. The grand parade of mountain peaks led us toward Glacier National Park. Once we reached White Fish, Montana, we stopped at an all-you-can-eat Pizza Hut.

After a 70 mile day, our bodies craved food. Hunger tugged at our minds. Does an all-you-can-eat joint affect you the way it does me? It makes me want to devour more than I need. When I was a kid, my dad used to take us out to the Marine Corps Thanksgiving and Christmas special base dinners. That was the one time of year when they set out the Ritz. We never went to a restaurant, so those two times of the year were special. Each time I stuffed myself so full, I got sick. To this day, when I go to an all-you-can-eat restaurant, I can't seem to stop until I make myself ill. The Pizza Hut was no different.

We stuffed every corner of our stomachs with pizza, salad bar goodies and apple strudel dessert. We ate and we ate some more. We kept eating. We got sick and we kept eating to get sicker. We suffered pain, but kept going back for more pain. That food meant more pain, but we couldn't stop.

"God, I'm sicker than a mule that just drank poison water and is carrying a 500 pound load," I said to Denis, rubbing my stomach. "I look like I'm six months pregnant."

He garbled in French a few moments and rolled his eyes.

"I think," he said, haltingly, "I have put too much in my mouth."

Even with that, we sat there looking at the blueberry strudel like a couple of kids in a candy store.

"One more time," I said.

Like being pulled on puppet strings, we slid out of the booth and headed back for more misery, more gluttony, and more pain. We found it, too.

Everyone looked as us, not believing the one dozen empty plates stacked up on our table. To knowingly make one's body sick like that means one must be sick in the head. Okay, we admit guilt. What ya' gonna' do? Arrest us? We were already so sick; we wished somebody would shoot us.

We paid the bill later and staggered into the darkening evening. To the west, the last rays of light played on the peaks, lighting them up like light bulbs, but that too was fading.

On Route 40, we headed straight toward Glacier. The sky turned pink, to orange, to shades of gray. We saw a gravel road leading up to an electrical house, fenced in, just above the highway. We popped the bikes into granny gear and cranked up to the top. Sure enough, it was a perfectly hidden flat spot, high above the highway. We saw cars from our perch, but they couldn't see us.

As Denis entered his tent, he said, "Four mosquitoes are in here waiting for me...no, make those four mosquitoes that no longer know life."

Our legs grew stronger, more powerful and with more endurance on uphill grades. We had done a few serious climbs the past couple of days. Soon, we'd be climbing the legendary "Road Going to the Sun."

How can traffic keep buzzing by at 3:00 and 4:00 in the morning? It's crazy for people to stay up and drive at all hours of the night. I slept well until I heard them roaring past on the highway below us. I stuffed my ears with plugs!

Nonetheless, we had to make 34 miles that day to camp at the base of the great climb to Logan's Pass. It would be an easy day.

Magnificent scenery, yes, with rolling highway and no steep up-hills! The bikes ran smoothly. We passed through Columbia Falls on a marginal road with no breakdown lane. That's where the old sphincters tightened as the big land yachts lumbered past, honking or cursing at us. Fat, rich, globby geezers in gas guzzling motor-homes scared the hell out of us by honking to push us over as they passed. Riding that road was like riding a tight rope at a circus. But we didn't have anywhere to go and no net. We watched five Prevost Greyhound-sized luxury motor homes go by dragging their five 4x4 Sport Utility Vans behind. They sported satellite dishes for their wide screen TV sets and a host of other toys. Those behemoths cost a quarter of a million dollars each and the vehicles behind were all $40,000.00. They stopped each night to hookups and electrics only to watch TV. Can't figure out why they spent so much to drive away from home just to watch the Nature Channel in a gravel-filled campground? They could have stayed home and done the same thing for nothing.

I swear to heaven that I will never travel in a motor-home even if I'm a millionaire. That's easy to say because my chances of becoming a millionaire are as probable as a mosquito flying to the moon on his own wing power.

While pedaling through small towns, I noticed flower displays in yards along the way. I decided to shoot a pictorial of Denis and his bike in front of the flowers. We took a shot of him at the end of a long line of flowers that curved around an intersection in Columbia Falls. Another shot came at a camping resort along the highway between Columbia Falls and Hungry Horse. Just before riding into Glacier, we took a shot of him near a restaurant sign with yellow flowers. During the ride, I made dozens of such shots and would turn them into a story for Adventure Cyclist Magazine.

After reaching Glacier visitor center, we stopped at the sign for pictures.

"It's nice to walk again," Denis said.

It was true. Our legs were used to pedaling seven to eight hours per day. Our quads hardened and our legs tightened. When walking, our legs felt spring loaded.

After paying our entrance fee, we rode along a two mile path through the woods to Apgar Village where we had to wait until 4:00 p.m. to ride the last 14 miles to Avalanche Lake. That would give us our best shot for riding to the top of Logan Pass by the 11:00 a.m. deadline. They tried to keep bikes off the roads at the peak hours.

"They ought to keep cars off the roads ALL the time," I said to the ranger.

"You know," he said. "I agree with you. They're seriously thinking about it at the Grand Canyon. They may start bus service here soon, too, and only allow walking or bike riding in the park."

"Good," I said. "It will promote more interaction with nature."

"You tell them mon ami," Denis quipped.

"Hrumph," I grunted, indignantly.

In the late afternoon, we pedaled along McDonald Lake for 11 miles. Ahead, we saw steep mountains and deep canyons. Beside us, the crystalline waters of the lake sparkled. Trees, mostly pine and aspen, grew along the shores, while rocky beaches invited us to stop, so we did. The road, full of cars, wound peacefully through dark green woods. Around 6:30 p.m., the warm air cooled and it was that magic hour when the balance in temperature held our bodies captive in its soothing grasp of not too hot and not too cool. We glided along in a perfect blend of speed, air, cranking and play. We felt fatigued from the day's ride yet powered by the easy rhythm of the slow pace.

At one point, the deep green woods on my left blew a cool jet of air out onto the road. It was as if someone had poured dry ice in a mist out to cool off tired bicycle travelers.

At 11 miles, the water ended and a road sign showed us how a glacier had formed the lake by advancing and then dumping a load of gravel at the terminus to block the melting water. Upon its retreat, a gorgeous blue lake formed.

Feeding it, a crystal clear river became our path upward. Every few miles it rushed down 50 foot falls much like the stairs to an old basement--turning it to white water. Riding along such incredible beauty made our pedaling an incidental unconscious function. I love it when riding becomes spiritual--where the body moves in a poetic, free-flowing, and effortless rhythm.

At Avalanche, we stopped in the Hiker-biker site. We fixed dinner and gobbled our food. A copy of a newspaper was left on the table. I picked it up.

"Good grief," I said to Denis. "Grizzlies mauled three people last week, and one guy fell off a cliff on the 'Going to the Sun Road.'"

"Did the others live?" he asked.

"Yup," I said. "But they're in a hospital from being clawed and chewed on."

"What were they doing to be attacked by a grizzly?"

"They were hiking, but one woman walked up on a mama grizzly and her cubs," I said. "The bear charged the lady and knocked her over a cliff...after that, the bear took her cubs and scrambled up the trail where she met two other hikers. She was surprised again and mauled them."

"What about the guy who died?"

"He stepped over the railing on the road and fell as he was taking a picture," I said.

"How do you say it in English?" Denis asked.

"Dumb shit," I said.

"That's it," Denis said.

Big red signs in the campground showed a ferocious grizzly growling at anyone who might read the warning. "You are in bear country. Make sure you keep your food locked in the trunk of your car and or lock boxes provided."

We brushed our teeth, washed our faces and placed our food bags into the lock box near the tents. No sense giving Mr. Grizz any reason to visit us for a midnight snack.

As I stood over the campfire brushing my teeth, I remembered the same signs in Alaska where I had traveled in the 80s. My brother Rex and I had made the big journey to the Land of the Midnight Sun. At one point, we camped on the Denali Highway just south of the McKinley National Park. In the morning, I awoke with a start. I heard some kind of animal outside my tent. I smelled it, something with a bad case of halitosis.

"Rex, you hear what I hear?" I whispered.

"Yeah, I can see him."

"What?"

"A grizzly."

I crawled out of my sleeping bag feeling a strange kind of fear welling up inside me. I felt like that once before when I was with a friend and he drove us into a near head-on accident. The pit of my stomach turned to acid and terror paralyzed me because I thought I was going to die.

Outside my tent at that moment, was another kind of death--something that I had admired from the distance the day before, but now, a wild creature, looking for food. It could be gentle and it might be savage. At that moment it could let us live or eat us, and we would not have much to say about it. Weighing in at 1,000 pounds or more, it was interesting to note that grizzlies make a living with their claws and teeth. I spied its brown fur right outside my tent flaps. I froze in place, not knowing what to do. I said nothing. Rex must have been thinking the same thing. Make no sounds and pray the beast left us in peace.

Seconds passed. I clutched my legs in pure fright as I squatted in the middle of the tent. Rex and I could live or die depending on the grizzly's appetite. Minutes passed as the big fellow grunted around our tents. I sat in a state of mental paralysis. My heart thundered against my ribs and I felt the blood racing through my arteries like Formula Ones carving around the turns at the Indy

500. Adrenaline dumped into my blood like someone had opened up a fire hydrant on a hot summer day. I wanted to escape, but my mind knew that a grizzly can outrun a deer for a short distance, so I squatted there.

They say your life passes before your eyes when you're about to die, but that wasn't true for me. I couldn't think of anything. Yet, I heard everything the bear did, DISTINCTLY! It dug around my tent, snorting and grunting. It sniffed the nylon and left a long trail of saliva across my roof. Five minutes passed as the bear worked its way around the end of my tent. Its shadow loomed across the nylon. That's when I heard a rip in the fabric at the back of my tent. I looked over my shoulder to see four long, black claws poking through the tan nylon of my fragile dwelling. Those claws measured four inches long! Dirt etched into the ends of them. Every cell in my body said, "RUN!" But my mind said, "STAY!" An instant later, the claws withdrew. The grizzly worked his way around to the front. His odor filled my lungs with fear. Soon, he dug for something ten feet away from my tent. I saw him through the crack in my tent flaps. Then something caught his attention in the brush and he ambled toward it. His dirty butt vanished into the bushes.

"Frosty," Rex whispered. "Are we going to live?"

"It's a toss up," I said. "We better keep calm so we don't attract his attention."

"I'm scared," Rex said.

"Shhhhh," I warned, still scared to death myself.

We waited for what seemed like an eternity before seeing the grizzly appear on a ridge a hundred yards away from us. He headed north without looking back. Mr. Grizz continued on about his life.

"Let's get the heck out of here," Rex said, as he crammed his sleeping bag into the stuff sack.

We broke camp in record time. While looking back over our shoulders, we made haste in the opposite direction.

That was a long time ago, but it was just like yesterday in my mind. Just thinking about it made my heart race. I gazed into the dying embers of the campfire. I thought how grand my life's good fortune, how lucky my star has been, how wondrous this great adventure of living.

"You have much to be thankful for," I muttered into the night air as I walked toward my tent.

I crawled through the zipper netting and into my warm sleeping bag. Denis snored a short distance away. I fell asleep for a long night's rest in my favorite place-- the wilderness.

The first robin hammered the morning air like a wrench hitting an anvil. In the east, the sun rose behind the great rock walls along Avalanche Creek. We broke camp as fast as possible--but didn't get out until 6:30.

We traveled beside the crystal waters of the river-- and through deep green woods. So green and silent we could hear only our derailleurs changing gears on the freewheels.

Only the rushing waters broke the quiet. Above us, huge vertical walls of rock with patches of snow, swept skyward. Green tundra patches spread across the mountains like a carpet laid by a master craftsman. From lofty places, snow fields dropped their load of freezing water into silver white cascades.

Every mile, we watched drops in the terrain create waterfalls resembling a bridal veil, at others, a sluice box of raging white water, and others dropped through rock crevasses like someone pouring coffee into a cup. Along with the white froth, a constant sound of rushing water echoed off the canyon walls.

We followed the road through the woods until we came upon a widening. The sun remained hidden, but rose over the crest of the mountains. The valley, still dark green in the shadows, lit up in a misty vapor trail streaming down from the notch in the summit. It was as if a spotlight shone down on a comedian through the smoke on the stage at some nightclub. But that spotlight came from 2,000 feet above! Such power it gave to our eyes....such spiritual wonder to our hearts.

The highway, a tiny sliver of asphalt, wove its way like a secretive snake through the deep forests until it began rising away from the river. Once away from the waters, it lifted like a 747 away from the canyon floor. Slowly our perspective changed as we gained altitude. The road took a hairpin curve to the right making us climb ever higher. We climbed along a narrow road with a rock wall rising a thousand feet on our left, and to our right, an expanse of pure mountain air. Breath-taking! Mesmerizing! Beguiling!

Each mile changed the view until we came back to a point perpendicular with the valley we had just pedaled up. Pink fireweed grew along the road on our right and we passed Heavens Peak at 8,800 feet. To our right, about a mile in the distance and 1,000 feet off the canyon floor, Bird Woman Falls dropped out of a hanging valley 492 feet to a ledge and sprayed in all directions as it made its way to the canyon floor. Thick snow fields fed the waterfalls, the most dramatic in the park. Upward we climbed from 3,000 to 4,000 to 5,000 feet.

We passed the "Weeping Wall" which offered a 40 yard long instant rain pouring out of a block of rock wall. We could have taken a shower with our biodegradable soap! The road construction crews preserved the wall when they built the road in 1936. Mr. George Grinnell was the superintendent of the park and had first set eyes on it in 1901.

At the time, he said, "Far away in northwestern Montana, hidden from view by clustering mountain peaks, lies an unmapped corner--the crown of the continent."

We kept pressing upward into the third hour. Ahead, the road continued along the flank of the mountain at a steady six percent grade. Upward still toward 6,000 feet, we labored. As we climbed, snowfields were no longer a distant sight, but level with us. What we had seen from the valley far below, we now saw from new angles and greater altitude. We were in the middle of what we saw from below. We had become a part of it.

We took great gulps of air from the waterfalls of Hatchet Creek that sprayed a cool mist onto us like air conditioning. At one point, the retaining wall on the cliff side had broken away and left a drop into nothingness. It was so sudden that it caused a gasp from Denis when he passed by it. The road was one a cyclist would not want to fall over. And if he did, he had better sprout wings quickly because it would be like jumping off the Empire State Building.

We could not imagine such raging white water mixed with snowfields that blended into tree-covered massive peaks. Each valley, cut as if with a razor sharp knife, offered astounding views. Jagged mountains, brown and bare at the top, swept downward into pine covered flanks and grassy flower-covered meadows. How did it feel cranking up a six percent grade for five hours? The pedaling became incidental as the splendor and the immensity of Glacier National Park swallowed us into its wonder and awe. Each rest stop/exhibit kept us constantly intrigued.

Into the fourth hour, and 13 miles, we saw the road zigzag to Logan's Pass. The cars ahead of us resembled ants making their way to the top. We pedaled past a snowfield that touched the road. The cold air coming off the snow cooled us. We made the last turn that swept upward past a waterfall--and over the top.

At the summit, an excellent visitor center gave folks a great view of the extraordinary features surrounding it. Cars and motor homes filled the parking lot. We arrived in late summer. We met two women who bicycled across America solo. Another had lost 40 pounds and was on a mission to prove herself. Another retired man pedaled from Maine. Another lady, Stacia, 21, pedaled in a 2,000 mile loop from Denver. She rode with a trailer behind her bike and a little teddy bear sitting on her handlebar bag. As we stood there, a parade of people walked by, some almost bewildered as to why we would attempt riding our bikes in such high places.

One retired guy said, "I feel sorry for you."

That's funny, because we touring cyclist revel in our energies, our lust for living and our challenges.

A natural amphitheater surrounded the center. Several trails gave visitors a chance to hike through snow-fields and on to high ridges. We grabbed our food bags and enjoyed a picnic along one of the walks. We gathered plenty of chipmunk company. A cool wind tugged at us at 6,600 feet. Yet, even where it was so cold, tiny tundra flowers in purple, pink, red and yellow opened their colors for all to see. They resembled tiny pin cushions specked with flowers. The sky, a brilliant liquid blue, profiled gray rock and aspirin-white snow. The Fuji film-colored green tundra rendered dramatic contrast. We drank in the view and stayed several hours to make sure we got our fill.

Dropping down the eastern side, we coasted downward through a mind boggling "U" shaped valley that stretched out of sight. A mantle of pines grew up one side--over the valley floor--and back up the other side like a loop in a roller coaster. Waterfalls poured down from the left and right with patches of snow creating a relief from all the green. Farther in the distance, brown layered peaks slanted upward with hundreds of levels of striations like a German chocolate cake with enough layers to reach 12,000 feet. And, above---nothing but sky! A.B. Guthrie named it "Big Sky." A cool wind blew in our faces.

We coasted down switchbacks to Jackson Glacier. We saw it from the road. The ranger said only 30 remained from the 137 they had noted at the turn of the century. Although a very short glacier, it impressed us with its size. It hung in a high valley across from us and looked like chocolate marble ice cream with its swirling layers of snow and rock. Most of the glaciers that cut the gargantuan peaks at Glacier National Park vanished with the last ice age--but their legacy remains a visual feast.

The road dropped for ten miles into trees, flowers, meadows and rivers. It was lined with cascading white water, rushing toward the valley floor. We kept burning our brake pads trying to keep our steeds from racing out of control.

Down we plunged like eagles--ever soaring on a velour, ribboned road. Where we had perched at the top of Logan's Pass, we now descended toward the far end of the valley where St. Mary's Lake collected all the water.

After the brake pads stopped burning, we pulled up at Sunrift Gorge. A short climb brought us to a narrow five foot cut in the layered rock where a raging trough of water raced downward--crashed into a rock wall--turned 90 degrees and raged again on its way to the valley floor. All the while, clear, clean, pristine misty cool vapors soothed our skin and lungs. Gees, isn't nature grand?!

Back on the road, we continued still high in the sky on our soaring flight downward until we reached the sparkling waters of St. Mary's Lake. We decided to camp at the Rising Sun Campground. When we stopped at the Hiker-biker site, we felt tired. I said to a camping neighbor, "Would you please cook dinner for us?"

"If you've got a blank check," he said. "I'll cook you up a seven course gourmet dinner."

"I was hopin' that anyone from Minnesota could fix up a home cooked meal but it looks like I can't afford you," I said.

"Well sir," he said. "I am a retired chef, but the operative word is 'retired.'"

Once again, Denis and I ate rice, beans, soup, bread, tea, hot chocolate and apples for dinner--just like we had for the past week. Food on a bike trip tastes like a New York chef's special every night! Hunger does amazing things to the mind.

Daylight crept over the mountains. We awoke among fellow campers fixing hot breakfasts. Eggs, bacon, hot coffee, yes, this was the great outdoors with our senses heightened to a wondrous level.

With the last six miles going down hill along St. Mary's Lake, we passed the Triple Divide Peak. Not prominent, but it was a peak where waters flowed east to the Atlantic, west to the Pacific and north into Hudson Bay.

In a twinkling, we rolled out of Glacier. Above us, big sky. In front of us, something new around the bend in the road ahead. Behind us, the second of our amazing five national parks reflected in our rear view mirrors.

"The little Rabbit sat quite still for a moment and never moved. He did not know the Fairy had kissed him and that had changed him forever. He found that he actually had back legs. Instead of dingy velveteen, he had brown fur, soft and shiny, his ears twitched by themselves, and his whiskers were so long that they brushed the grass. He gave one leap and the joy of those legs was so great that he went springing about the turf on them, jumping sideways and whirling round as the others did, and he grew so excited that when at last he did stop to look for the Fairy, she was gone."

The Velveteen Rabbit
Margery Williams

Motels dotted East Glacier. That's all it was—a series of motels. We bought some food and saddled up. The road out of town swept upward toward a distant pass. We couldn't see much at first, but soon, glorious views of the park spread before us like a visual horn of plenty.

Struggling mightily up an eight percent grade, we reached the top at noon. Lunch under a stand of pines gave us renewed energy. From the pass, we watched the road ribbon off into the distance along the east side of the Continental Divide. Down we flew into the valley. Soon, we rolled up and down over hill and dale until reaching Kiowa Junction.

The road flattened, and for once we settled into a steady pace going straight ahead. I fell in back of Denis and watched his freewheel for awhile...the grade changed and he deftly shifted into a lower gear...the chain climbed up the cogs and settled into its new route. I did the same. Denis' legs pounded like pistons and his feet feathered the ground. I looked at my own legs, and like pistons, they too, pounded up and down in a constant rotation of power and release, power and release. I rolled quietly behind Denis as he set the pace and cut through the air. We imitated two geese on a flight south...the lead goose plowed the wind to give his friends time to rest.

Soon, Denis dropped back and I took the lead. It was harder, but I felt a greater purpose to give my friend a break from the wind. Sweat poured down from my chin and splashed on the top tube. My shirt soaked up. Sweat ran down my back. My neck glistened. My legs powered me forward in a steady rhythm of perfection.

Bicycle 'satori' becomes a point where body, mind and spirit flow into unconsciousness of being. In that zone, there is no past, present or future. No worry or concern! No yes or no! Just being! I dropped into that state for miles ahead of and behind Denis. When behind him, all I could 'see' was his freewheel turning. When in front, I saw nothing but the pavement rushing past in a blur. Nothing mattered. Time did not exist. I moved with constant power and release, rotation and repeat, sweat drops and sunshine.

The Indian village of Browning stood like an outpost on the plains where the once mighty Blackfeet ruled the land. Where they hunted the buffalo and enjoyed their lives, they now exist on a reservation. Ironic enough, in only 80 years after dozens of tribes of Indians helped the Louis and Clark Expedition through that area on their way to the West Coast in 1803, the white man slaughtered an estimated eight million Indians, and by 1880, forced them onto reservations and gave them whiskey along with religion.

They haven't recovered and never will.

The famous bronze statues by Bob Scriver greeted us near the Plains Indian Museum. Scriver depicted bucking broncos with riders reaching for the sky. His renditions of buffaloes and Indians astound one's eyes. It's amazing that bronze possesses so much feeling in the hands of a master sculptor.

While loading our food from the market, two drunken Indians walked up to me and asked for money. I shook my head. They turned and left. But they made a terrible impact on me. Once mighty warriors--the white man destroyed their culture. Where they galloped across the plains, they now stooped into liquor and the use of a thing called "money." There were 522 Indian tribes when settlers arrived in America. Today, Indians live on reservations in America, and for the most part, the white man ruined and destroyed their cultures. They have not and do not mesh with present-day modern society. They are stuck in an in-between world of a collective anachronism. And, there is nothing that can be done to make it better.

We caught a tailwind out of town and it blew us for the next 20 miles of easy riding over a grass-lined road as flat as a pancake on a Saturday morning griddle. Pour a little hot maple syrup along with some melted butter and you've got yourself a perfect smooooooooth ride. No trees existed for as far as the eyes could see--only waving brown grasses undulating to the horizon. Every once in awhile, a rabbit hopped through the bush.

"More big wind please," Denis said.

"As long as it's behind us," I said.

Late in the afternoon, I wanted to camp in back of an old rock quarry, but Denis talked me into the ride to Depuyer.

We rode along some fresh asphalt on a smooth flat strip of land between fields of barley. The sun sank lower in the sky--my butt hurt--and I was tired. My butt really hurt as we neared Depuyer. It felt like someone had taken a paddle and spanked me. About three miles out of Depuyer, our shadows stretched 20 yards across the highway to the east. We rode as two shadows on a lonely road with four legs pounding the pedals and our shadows following our every move. The first of the thunderheads popped up and swirled like cotton candy. The sunlight fringed the clouds in fiery glory like a raging fire searing and scorching across the liquid blue sky.

About 7:45 p.m., we rode nine miles out of Depuyer. Denis wanted to go into the town for a camp spot. I wasn't thrilled about pedaling another 45 minutes just to get into town. He kept pressing me, but my heart wasn't into it. As darkness descended, I was like a mule that wouldn't budge. We rode beside a river flowing perpendicular to the road.

"Denis," I said. "Let's camp here. My legs are tired and my butt is killing me."

"Let's make Depuyer," he said.

"I don't want to ride in the dark," I said, pulling over to two dirt tracks leading off the road and beside the river.

"We could reach a picnic table in town," he said.

"You go ahead," I said. "I'll catch you in the morning."

With that Denis reluctantly turned, and we found a spot 40 yards off the road near the river. It was out in the middle of nowhere. I liked that location. As we got off the bikes, a mine field of cowpies confronted us--big, brown, piles of cow shit. It was like trying to play hopscotch as we moved the bikes and ourselves toward the flat spots for the tents. Unfortunately, cowpies dotted the area on all sides of us. I found a place in the middle of four cowpies, but right in the middle of my front door opening was a giant cowpie. Must have been a bull for it was a pile of dung that rivaled a pitcher's mound in pro baseball. Scared me, the smell that is. My tent popped up as the sky turned to fire.

The sun began its fiery egress from the day. Far off to the west, blazing streaks of light burst from the burning globe of the sun like the prongs off the Statue of Liberty. Columns of light sprayed across the sky--first in gold and quickly turning to strawberry red. On the eastern horizon, battleship-sized thunderheads stacked up like mashed potatoes being dumped from heaven. As they packed themselves across the sky, each thunderhead burst with red, crimson and gray in the deep pockets of its rumbling mist. Just as suddenly, a half moon appeared through the clouds and shone like someone burning a single flashlight in the sky.

With a silent piercing last cry, the sun vanished. The long flat clouds near the western horizon began burning on their edges in bright fire engine red tones of reflected light. All the while, the river beside our campsite rippled and gurgled with the current. While this magnificent color display raged across the sky, we pitched our tents and set up our sleeping bags with air mattresses spread out. While this silent symphony heralded the coming of the night, we cooked dinner on the flat ground.

As the soup steamed, the sky changed to yet another reddened hue. When the pasta softened, the sun continued on its way across the Pacific leaving one, then two and finally a dozen stars twinkling above us. By the time we got to the hot chocolate, the sky spoke not a word in colors but had turned into ink black space... dotted with a silvery moon and a zillion stars. We didn't have to look up because we felt our place on the ancient Indian Blackfoot plains was the grandest grandstand for watching the universe do its thing. It's been said that sunshine brings flowers and that God's laughter is their blooming. But the night must be God's slumber because on the plains out in the middle of nowhere, it was so quiet; we heard the pulse of the universe. We sat there, campfire embers jumping and sizzling, watching the Big Dipper pour its magic into our souls.

Sublime.

CHAPTER 6 — FRYING PAN FULL OF FEAR

"We travel through the voids of space on a small, self-contained life vessel powered by the energy of the stars. It is a marvelous ship of life, probably one of the most wondrous and rare in the universe. Yet, in our human centered ignorance and arrogance, we have tried to create a different world, to confine the other species that share the vessel with us to smaller and smaller compartments while we command more and more space for our burgeoning numbers and desires. The earth is in danger of becoming a monstrous slave ship sailing on the cosmic tides of the Milky Way. To support our expanding population of human passengers we are systematically destroying or enslaving much of the other life of the ship we sail upon. And we have used the fossil sunlight and water discovered in various holds of the ship to support artificial compartments where a relatively small number of us live in amazing luxury. In fact, compared to the majority of the ship's human passengers most of us in western societies live in these synthetic, unnatural settings like swollen grubs feeding

off the energy-rich micro-environments we have created,
all the while spewing forth our resulting disorder and
poisonous wastes to contaminate other areas of the vessel.
What's even worse is that we add 85 million of us each
year to this ever diminishing vessel called earth--our
planet home."

Steve Van Matre

That night, I awoke twice with a sudden jolt thinking I had landed full body in the middle of a giant pile of cow dung. Fortunately only coyote howls carried across the prairie. We camped in the middle of nowhere--which for a time in life was a good place to be. We had named the place "Camp Cowpie."

Depuyer turned out to be a nice little nothing of a town where Lewis, of Lewis and Clark, traveled back through on his way to St. Louis. A grass field with toilets and picnic tables awaited us at the end of town. Had I not been such a wussy, sissy, crybaby, whiner, groaner and complainer—we could have enjoyed civilized picnic tables and a place to park our butts in the bathrooms. Of course, we would have heard dogs barking, cat fights, the click of the night sprinkler system, and a couple of drunks who left their twelve packs on one of the tables. Nothing like a conversation with a couple of drunks--stimulating, enthralling and captivating.

Drunks share a particular world that escapes me having never been drunk in my life. In college, I saw them first--upchuck their dinner and once the contents of their stomachs vanished, they continued with the 'dry' heaves for hours until their bodies writhed in pain from the muscle contractions and nothing left to heave forward. They repeated that regimen week after week. I never figured out why it was more fun than racquetball, tennis, dancing with the girls and/or kissing them.

Nonetheless, Denis gave me a stern lecture about why we should have made the little park in Depuyer. I got down on my knees and begged for his forgiveness. Next time, I would be brave and forget my weariness, my aching butt, my tired bones and my personal suffering. Next time, I would keep pedaling and reach the "Promised Land." After lots of begging, he granted forgiveness with a sly smile.

Denis proved light hearted and prone to making jokes. I chuckled many times on the trip. Physically, I tried to keep up with him, but his legs out-powered mine. John Brown was the same way. I remember him on our 1986 coast-to-coast bicycle adventure when a 21 year old college kid challenged John. Kevin, the kid, ended up with a damaged Achilles tendon and had to walk up long grades in order to stay with our ride across America.

In Texas, one rather hot day, I too tried to show my legs possessed more power by trying to beat John. We rode 10 miles out of a small town named Clairborne. While pedaling along, we never said a word, but the race started with a simple challenge of pressing the pedals down a bit faster. Soon, we flew down the highway under a hot Texas sun. I cranked the pedals with all my might.

I grabbed a lead on John, but he kept hanging in there. By the time we were three miles out of the town, my legs burned, my saliva thickened like molasses in autumn, and my lungs burned from sucking in so much air. I knew if I could hold on the last mile, I'd 'win' the race. But at the end, John powered up his legs and blasted past me. I didn't stand a chance. Just a bit of friendly testosterone between friends!

Now, 10,000 miles away, he sat in bed with a chemo drip stuck in his arm. Funny how life changes for anyone so quickly. One moment you're about to retire and go on a bicycle adventure; the next, you've got cancer. Hard to figure out how life chooses some of us to live and some of us to suffer, and/or die.

Denis and I stopped at the store in Depuyer. A rusted 1928 McCormick-Deering tractor was parked along the highway. Later, we rode through another small town named Bynum. It featured turn-of-the-century buildings. One resident had filled a manure wagon with flowers. For the most part, those small towns filled with people who enjoyed a simple life. They also didn't mind junk lying everywhere in town or their yards. Mostly, things were broken down, decaying and ugly.

In Choteau, the town featured a fabulous museum of dinosaurs, old gas pumps, and human skeletons of men who had been hanged or shot with arrows. A.B. Guthrie, the author of "Big Sky" played a prominent role in the area as he had been a resident before his death.

We buzzed through Mayfair into a steady head wind on Route 87/89. But the road turned on us and like a miracle, we enjoyed tailwinds that blew us into Great Falls, Montana. There's nothing like a tailwind. It lifted our spirits and we smiled from ear to ear. We pedaled easily on a flat, well-paved road. Traffic was light. Have I mentioned how much I love a tailwind? This one proved a honey of a wind and we enjoyed every hour of it sweeping us down the highway as if we were powered by an engine.

Lewis and Clark Interpretive Center proved one of the best exhibits I've ever seen concerning our country's history of the West. That museum brought the entire expedition of 1804—06 into living perspective. I read about it in history books as a kid.

I crossed the Lewis and Clark Trail a dozen times in my travels across America. But not until the day we stopped into the newly opened center did I have any idea what a monumentally dangerous journey they pursued and survived.

The co-commanders on the trip were Meriwether Lewis, the boyhood friend of Thomas Jefferson, and William Clark who accepted their positions on what Jefferson described as an exploration to find a river passage out of the Louisiana Purchase to the Pacific. The two young men were well educated, resourceful, frontiersmen, Army officers and courageous. Their journey marked a blend of raw adventure and scientific investigation for a growing nation filled with expectation.

The Lewis and Clark Expedition proved one of the most dramatic and significant episodes in the history of the United States. It stands as America's epic exploration of the American West. In 1804, it carried the destiny as well as the flag of our nation westward from the Mississippi River to the Pacific Ocean. It fired the imagination of the American people. We still read about it today and celebrate the trail.

At the time, the purchase of the territory doubled the size of America. Thomas Jefferson wanted to lay claim to the newly acquired land, which he bought at two cents an acre from Napoleon, and gain a foothold for America all the way to Oregon. With that vision, he created "The Corps of Discovery."

Both Lewis and Clark excelled in many skills--map making, navigation, survival in the wilds, leadership, horticulture, geology and other sciences. They set off from St. Louis in May of 1804 and headed up the Missouri River. The party numbered 45 men, a slave named York, and a Newfoundland dog named Seaman. The men forced their keelboats up the treacherous river waters. They dragged them for days with ropes from the shore. Their hands blistered and bled. One man died.

The first of many councils with Indian tribes occurred near Omaha, Nebraska, which is why Council Bluffs was so named. Clark gave presents and medals to Oto chiefs and informed them of the new sovereignty of the United States. Little did the chiefs know they would get their butts shot off in the following years and their lands stolen.

The expedition spent the winter in what is now North Dakota. They traded with the Mandan and Minitari Indians. They recruited a French fur trader named Toussaint Charbonneau and his wife, Sacagawea, to guide them west over the Rockies.

They came through Great Falls in June of 1805 and spent three weeks portaging their heavy canoes up the rapids some 18 miles around the falls. They reached the Shoshoni Indians, where, if it had not been for Sacagawea knowing the leader who was her brother, the entire party would have been killed. Leave it to a woman to save a bunch of pale faces!

They trudged further west on the Clearwater, Snake and finally, the mighty Columbia River until they reached the Pacific. During their journey, they nearly starved to death and suffered grizzly attacks, mountain lions and bugs. Indians stole their horses and supplies. After reaching the Pacific, they stayed the winter. Not being able to catch a ship around the Cape, they had to push back up the Columbia eastward toward home.

The Corps traded their canoes for pack horses and traversed the Rocky Mountains a second time. In July 1806, they reached current day Missoula, Montana. The party split and explored two different routes back to St. Louis. On the way, they killed a couple of Indians which became the first of millions. They raced back home and on September 23, 1806, they returned to the cheering crowds on the docks of St. Louis. The expedition had covered 8,000 miles in two years, survived starvation, disease, heavy snows, and wild animals.

For anyone who wants a truly unique day of history, this place is superb. I loved it. It filled in a lot of blank spots in my understanding of the expedition. Denis and I watched a movie that made the Trail and men come alive. Afterward, a route through the center showed how the Indians saved Lewis and Clark's lives, gave them food and guidance, as well as horses and canoes. Those guys proved tougher than a bunch of Navy Seals, Green Berets and Marines. They lived by their wits.

Later in the day, we caught a tailwind for 24 miles to the junction of 87/89 to Monarch. We stopped at a roadside rest area with covered tables.

As I sit here at this picnic table, the sky blazes 1950s-shower stall pale blue tile with thin white clouds streaking the heavens like someone had slashed it with a machete--and to the west the sun boils into a low lying cloud bank. Nature once again works its magic all around me. The day has passed and I am blessed again with an exquisite life. How many men my age, or any age get to ride their bicycle across the country? As old age creeps into me like a piece of gnarled wood being weathered by the years in the sun, I will continue in my youthful ways for as long as life lets me. And when I can't, I will check out on my terms. No rest home where we sit around and play cribbage. No letting Alzheimer's disease take me down slowly and miserably. No dinner hour where we gather at the same table to eat the same mundane food. No meaningless banter about someone's daughter or son's accomplishments. Screw that! No sitting for hours watching a game show or someone else living it up. I'm going to suck the marrow out of life's body. On my last day, I'll be worn out, used up and ready for my last ride.

In many ways, our lives are like Lewis and Clark's expedition. We have a beginning where we don't know what's going to happen. We wonder what's out there. Our curiosity, much like a cat's, is piqued by the books we read or the TV Nature Channel. Maybe we met a character who told us a story about some place he had seen. Or, our parents took us on a trip and our appetites became whetted by the experience. With each day, as we grow into our 20s, life pulls us outward--toward our destiny. Many choose safety and security. Others choose danger and uncertainty.

Me? I choose the unknown. Is it dangerous? Perhaps. Will it kill me? Maybe. For me, life is an evolutionary trek through time. Like that bear who has no idea when he or she will die, I too live each day with an expectation of my potential. As long as I'm not dying or dead, I'm alive and enjoying the ride. My old friend Napoleon Hill said, "There are two ways of relating one's self to life: One is that of playing horse while Life rides. The other is that of becoming the rider while Life plays horse. The choice as to whether one becomes the horse or the rider is the privilege of every person, but this much is certain: if one does not choose to become the rider of Life, he is sure to be forced to become the horse. Life either rides or is ridden. It never stands still."

Nor do I. My grandmother used to say I burned the candle at both ends and I would burn out long before I was supposed to. What she didn't realize was that my candle is SOOOO LONNNGGG! At least I think it's long. It must be attitude.

The sky took a turn to cheap bordello pink with a few feathered clouds that would make a Las Vegas show girl proud.

We ate dinner. As we cleaned the pans, Denis said, "Have you seen my can opener?"

"I already put mine away," I said, rattling my mess kit.

"There was salmon on it," he said. "I worry about grizzlies smelling it and paying us a late night visit."

"There aren't any grizzlies around here," I said. "So, you don't have to worry."

"Just on postcards?" Denis said.

"Yes," I said, smiling. "Only on postcards."

"We sure have it better than Lewis and Clark," he said.

"Yeah," I said. "But I think we were born 200 years too late."

"No," he said. "We're exploring just like they did."

"You're right," I said. "This is our time and we're making the best of it."

Chapter 7 — Life Means Movement

"Mountains should be climbed with as little effort as possible and without desire. The reality of your own nature should determine the speed. If you become restless, speed up. If you become winded slow down. You climb the mountain in equilibrium between restlessness and exhaustion. Then, when you're no longer thinking ahead, each footstep isn't just a means to an end, but a unique event in itself. "This" leaf has jagged edges. "This" rock looks loose. From "this" place the snow is less visible, even though closer. These are things you want to notice anyway. To live only for some future goal is shallow. It's the sides of the mountains which sustain life, not the top."

Robert Pirsig

"You didn't tell me about the sprinkler factor," Denis said in the morning.

"I didn't think about it," I said. "How would I know about sprinklers?"

"So why did you put your tent on the cement and away from the grass?" he asked.

"Too lazy to push in the stakes," I said.

Denis rolled his eyes and threw up his hands. My tent was on the cement and under the roof of our small pavilion. Denis pitched his tent in the grass. During the night, the sprinkler system kicked on and soaked his tent plus made a splashing sound until he moved it. The same thing happened at a former campsite in one of the city parks where we had camped.

Not only that, a train roared through at 3:00 a.m., sounding like it was headed for our front doors. Now there is an interesting feeling having a train run through your brain in the middle of the night. Diesel trucks rolled through and popped their air brakes in the parking lot. I crammed a pound of toilet paper into my ears so I didn't hear so much of the noise.

While cooking our oatmeal, Don and Melinda, 70 year old newly-weds stopped to talk with us. They marveled that we had the health to ride bikes across the country. Don's knees were shot and he was lucky to ride his bike around the block. However, for newlyweds, they felt excited about their lives together. Cher once said in an interview that, "Like grass growing through old cracks in the pavement, love can grow into people at any age."

Don and Melinda represented that passionate look!

We cranked along a river up Route 89 against a strong 20 mph head wind. We enjoyed a smooth highway while riding beneath rock cliffs with trees along our route as well as sparkling river water. At the end of the valley, we climbed two hours up a steep grade to roll over a pass. There's something about busting your butt on a steep climb of eight to 10 percent grade. At first, it looks impossible, but you head into it one revolution at a time. Soon, the valley floor fades away with more altitude. On the way up, large vistas open to newer perspectives of the land. Your body sweats, drips on the top tube, your hair gets sweaty wet, your nose drips with sweat and a small stream runs down the middle of your back. Your gloves soak up. Even your ears sweat. It's hard work cranking up a mountain pass road. At the top, the grade lessons and your body feels the ease in the muscle expenditure. You shift into higher gears as the road flattens. Moments later, it's a 'free' gravity powered ride. Down, down and down you go...coasting through the turns, rounding the curves, gaining speed and loving the feeling of free flight. It brings such a delight to the mind. Amazingly enough, I never think about the climb because it just is what it is.

At the top, the road plunged back into a canyon. I followed Denis at high speed. About five miles into our gravity powered descent, a loud bang erupted from Denis' back tire. His rear end slipped sideways like an Indy 500 race car out of control on a curve. Denis touched the brakes lightly but the beast beneath him continued on its wild bucking motion.

His eyes grew as big as eggs 'easy over', while a frying pan full of fear gripped his heart. One wrong move could catapult him over the bars and face first on the unforgiving asphalt. He feared for his handsome face. Every muscle in his body tightened and his sphincters, already working overtime with the dilemma facing them, or would that be better said, in back of them, tightened into an eternal rectal kiss. This was no time for laughter or levity. He had to keep his iron stallion upright and prepare to leap, like one of those old stage drivers, if it went down.

His speed dropped from 40 to 30, 20 and 10. He touched the brakes gently until the bike slowed to a stop. He looked down to see that the metal rim had separated from itself.

Off to the side of the road, we surmised that his mountain bike had been ridden for so long and the brakes had been applied so many times in the dirt, that the rim had worn thin and finally collapsed under the load and the speed of his ride down the hill.

He pulled off the gear and detached the wheel. Sure enough, the metal rim suffered separation. It split alongside where the brake pad had worn it over a period of time. Metal fatigue! Denis, being an excellent bike rider, saved his butt from road rash, cuts and possible death by his deft handling of his wounded steed.

"This wheel almost killed my life," he said.

"No kiddin'," I said. "Glad I wasn't following you too closely or I would have run right up your rear end."

"I must go back to Great Falls for a new rim," he said.

"Let's hitch a ride into Monarch and find a ride back to Great Falls," I said.

Denis flagged a ride from a guy named Joe in a pickup truck. I followed into Monarch, a little one-horse mountain town, where I asked around for someone heading to Great Falls. A couple of Air Force sergeants decided to give Denis a lift.

They took him to the Shields Bike shop in Great Falls. I remained with his gear. Luckily, the restaurant offered a little bar and seats. I sat in air-conditioned comfort for the next six hours. I read Abbey's "Desert Solitaire" the whole time.

The event reminded me of the time when John Brown had leveraged up his bike with his feet against the rims near Death Valley on our 1986 coast-to-coast ride. In a split second, he turned his rim into a pretzel. It looked as if a Mack truck ran over it. In the blink of an eye, he trashed his traveling machine, kaput, toast--a hurtin' hunk of metal. In other words, he really screwed himself.

After standing out in the middle of 100 plus degree heat, we flagged down a tourist who sold John a new rim from his own bike hanging off his car. We were so excited to have our mobility back, especially in that deadly place. Even rattlers and lizards breathed hard in the desert, so you can imagine how we felt. We pedaled up Panamint Valley on our way over the pass into Death Valley. We were so happy to have his wheel working, we burst in song, "It's a good day for singin' a song and it's a good day for ridin' along, and it's a good day for singin' a song, yes, it's a good day for ridin' our bikes...oh we're singing and pedaling along, yes singin' and pedaling along...." Mind you, our voices were not Elvis Presley or Ray Orbison. More like a couple of coyotes drunk on peyote!

That night, we slept by the sign, "Welcome to Death Valley", in a howling windstorm. The stars came out and it was a good time in our lives. So often in my life, bad things have happened, big and small, and each time, my attitude turned the event into a positive. John Brown is the same way. That's why I love the man. There is a song, "Always look on the bright side of life, always look on the bright side of life...." Whoever wrote it expressed brilliance.

As I sat there, John's cancer condition weighed heavy on my mind. He battled daily with vomiting and nausea from chemo while we sweated up mountain passes. We struggled up passes while he fought for his life. It's not a funny or fun battle. Lance Armstrong, the great American rider who won the Tour de France seven times, struggled against horrific odds too, and won. However, when it comes to cancer, it's a crap shoot. Much like Armstrong, John's invincible spirit played a roll. I could only imagine both these men winning from sheer tenacity and love of life.

Several hours later, Denis returned with a new rim. He had hitched with two people to make it back. We put the rim on the bike and rode south toward Yellowstone.

After two weeks on the tour, my legs felt strong and powerful. My thighs felt like two springs coiled under the skin. The muscles responded to hills without hesitation. My lungs grew stronger in their ability to pull all the oxygen I needed to power my body down the road.

I stretched during breaks as well as did pushups in my tent at night. My bike, named Condor for the high places he had taken me in Asia, North and South America, felt smooth under my saddle. He became a part of my body.

Late in the afternoon, a half dozen hawks played tag with themselves by flying from fence post to fence post along the road. The land undulated for miles in front us. Later a group of swallows flitted in the breezes that swirled everywhere. Grasses waved and bent along the highway as we pressed onward. Flowers captured my attention at every turn in the road--red, yellow, white and purple. Each time we crossed a river, its cool air refreshed me. Above, the sky displayed its cloud magic. Sometimes, they resembled marching soldiers on high, and at others, they painted feather wisps on the blue canvas of the universe. During storms, they rolled in like a gray layer cake that hung low to the ground. But the most powerful shapes were the thunderheads that boiled upward into the heavens like Mount Saint Helens erupting. On calm days, they stood still and on windy days they skittered across the sky like nervous birds. Sometimes, an oval spaceship-shaped-cloud hovered above us. In the morning none existed, but by noon, a single cloud gathered above. By evening, that cloud beckoned his buddies who gathered around as if awaiting the sun's final body painting party. On the western plains, it rarely disappointed. At 12 mph, the world passed by deliberately, quietly, peacefully--spiritually.

What does spirituality mean on a bicycle? For me, it feels like I'm closer to the rhythms of nature--of life itself. My pace allows my senses to absorb and enjoy my surroundings. My spirit meshes, like raindrops on a field of wildflowers, with the forces of life. Better yet, like a seal slipping through the water, as she plays at living. I too play at life and feel fulfilled, peaceful and happy inside.

Conversely a book by Ishak Bentov titled: "STALKING THE WILD PENDULUM" describes what happened to western man because he/she stepped outside the "circle of life." He says everything in the universe vibrates...water, air, rock, fire, wind, all creatures--everything.

Everything 'dances' to the rhythms of the universe. Unfortunately, humans have ensconced themselves into concrete cities. They walk on asphalt and look through glass and live in square buildings. Humans no longer forage for food or fight or flight. (Except when they battle for hot dogs at an NFL football game where they lust for the savagery on the field!)

Many humans in industrialized countries work at jobs that have no meaning in their lives or spirits. Instead of birds, thunder, lightning and winds for sound, they suffer acid rock and heavy metal blasting through their eardrums. Horns, lights and train whistles tell them what to do.

They travel in steel and glass containers called cars and they suffer road rage or crawl into pills like Advil to take away the pain. In short, humans in industrialized societies exist out of tune with nature and themselves.

Those who can, travel to the lakes, hills, mountains or rivers on weekends to camp out, hike or ski. They essentially move among nature's wonders and "re-tune" their spirits and bodies, which refreshes them. They get a dose of 'nature' instead of Prozac. For those who don't or can't-- they drink, smoke, do other drugs, eat too much, shop till they drop, watch hockey violence, NFL, Smack-Down wrestling or boxing. Many space out on the boob tube. Many go about life in various degrees of mental instability.

I wish I could help everyone follow their dreams--to pursue their passions, to "go where the brave dare not go... to fight the unbeatable foe." I'm not saying it's easy, but I'm saying that anyone can choose their quest--and succeed at it. When I think of the 100 hour work weeks I worked busting my butt for 20 summers in an 18-wheeler, breaking my back and mind moving heavy furniture...well, it wasn't easy. But, it got me to my dreams of world adventure. No one can say that I've been lucky or had it easy. I never gave up my dreams. Not now, not ever!

Why am I successful? Simple! I created 'intentions' that I planted into the quantum field of the universe.

Once planted with my thoughts, those ideas took root like corn takes root in a field. I cultivated my dreams until they sprouted into reality. From that point, I made my ideas live as actions.

When it comes to free time, I wish I could tell the world how incredible it is to take a bicycle ride, if only for a day or weekend!

Talk about being in rhythm with life! To feel my body work, struggle and succeed is a life-giving endeavor. Sure, it takes work! That's what the body loves. I never want to be too comfortable. I'll shoot myself before I travel in a motor home! I must quest with a thundering heart, pounding, even gasping for oxygen as I crank up a mountain toward the top. It's not the destination, but power and involvement in the journey that interest me more than comfort and ease. I relish the struggle.

By 6:00 p.m., we pedaled down the highway along Crawford Creek--a lazy, knee deep, slow moving stream with king fishers flying along its rock strewn surface. The sun left us in the shadows and the fresh cool air coming off the stream delighted our skin and noses. For a half hour, we felt the change from the heat of the day to the cool of the evening. The flat road, the still air, the spinning spokes, the shadows playing on the mountain flanks, the rushing sound of water over small falls, and the deep silent forest along both sides of the road--all made for magic for our ride into the twilight.

By 8:00 p.m., we pedaled into a riverside campsite. After two days of sweat that had dried a dozen times and soaked me over and over, I was about as close to my animal ancestors, probably Neanderthals, in body odor as I could get. I hardly breathed without choking myself. I needed a bath.

"Tu ai un grand gross odor," Denis muttered when he neared me.

"I heard that," I said. "I need a dip in the stream."

But that was a problem in a river that was running off snowfields. This would be an ice cube bath. Should a bath cause pain? Is it fair to make every skin cell on your body break down in tears...pleading for mercy? Can it be good to make your body shiver and moan in agony? Is causing oneself pain a sort of masochistic endeavor? Would it be worth it? YES! If you want to be clean!

Oh my God, but that first dip under the water was a shrill thrill. I screamed. Every cell on my skin curled back like the soldiers in Custer's Last Stand. My shrill cry pierced the quiet woods.

Denis raced over to me, "Are you okay?"

"No!" I said. "I'm freezing my patootie off...what does it look like...I'm having a good time in a hot springs?"

I soaped up, biodegradable, of course, and had to rinse off with a pan 30 feet from the water. It took me three trips and nearly killed me as I poured frigid streams of water down my head and over my shoulders. It was like icy knives carving my body up like bacon strips.

Suddenly, I rinsed clean. Heavenly feeling!

We ate a dinner of rice, bell peppers, lentils, bread, tea and noodle soup. I broke out the hot chocolate.

Later we sat by a warm campfire. With a clear night sky, the stars sifted through the leaves in the trees overhead. A full moon followed. Silver bright and just right. We sat by the fire--flames licking upward into the darkness. I loved the peacefulness the flames gave my mind.

They vanquished any labored thoughts.

"This is the answer," I said, bringing my rock closer to the fire to sit on.

"This is nice," Denis said, flattening his palms toward the fire. "I really liked seeing that king fisher fly ahead of us along the river."

"Seemed like he was leading us to this campsite," I said.

"There is much to be learned from our fellow travelers," Denis said, throwing more wood onto the fire.

"Indeed there is!"

CHAPTER 8 — KEEP PEDALING FOREVER

"All great teachers have preached that man, originally, was a "wanderer in the scorching and barren wilderness of this world....to rediscover his humanity, he must slough off attachments and take to the road."

Dostoyevsky

"Our nature lies in movement; complete calm is death."

Rene Pascal

"For me, the question of questions: the nature of human restlessness."

Bruce Chatwin

"Drifting about among flowers and sunshine, I am like a butterfly or bee, though not half so busy or with so sure an aim. But in the midst of these methodless rovings I seek to spell out by close inspection things not well understood."

John Muir

Down the road, I must read more Emerson, Paine, Edison, Darwin, Lincoln, Burbank, Napoleon, Ford, Carnegie, Muir, Steinbeck, Milton, Sartre, Mills, Twain, London, Bach, Dickens, Jefferson, Einstein, Rand, Stegner, Leopold, Socrates, Aristotle, Plato...and the list goes on.

At the age of 52, it has dawned on me that there is not enough time to live this life. I can't get to those minds fast enough through their books. But I do know that I have to keep moving--discovering what they discovered in my own way. Their trek is now my trek. What is the most amazing thing about this life journey? I think it's the direction each of us chooses. For anyone not gouging out a rut in their daily living, a person can create anything and do anything. Picasso took a wild ride. So did Jim Morrison. One was long and one very short. Did it make any difference at the point of their deaths? Probably! One enjoyed enduring satisfaction for lust realized in the art form expressed for many years.

For Morrison, a flame turned up to high temperatures and a quick flame out. Too bad...not even a wrinkle or gray hair. Never that thing called wisdom. I think it is much better to be tired of living from SO much living than to check out with only a taste on the tip of my tongue. In fact, I'd like to be so full of living that I am weary of breathing and can't wait to be gone. Time and fate will tell. Who orchestrates it? Any guess will do. I once read, "Life is not a journey to the grave with the intention of arriving safely in a pretty and well-preserved body, but rather to skid into home plate broadside, thoroughly used up, totally worn out and loudly proclaiming, 'Wow! That was a hell of a ride!'"

We pedaled into Neihart, a former mining town, with at one time, 4,000 back-broken souls, and for their masculine delight, a bordello. As we neared the village, old mining ruins stood along the highway. It's always discouraging to me that the people who gained riches and wealth from the mines leave their trash, oil drums, buildings and junk behind when they have exhausted the resources.

Many buildings I photographed were constructed in the 1880s. I talked to one 75 year old lady running the grocery store and she said the building I wanted to photograph was a livery stable from 1895. It featured a rusted, galvanized steel roof that was so old, its sides waved like a ribbon in the wind. I took a picture with the bike in front. The brown wood had cracked in so many places, and light streamed into the building like laser swords in Star Wars. Also in Niehard was a junk dealer who wrote on his building, "This ain't no museum. I've got junk for sale. Don't forget, I buy junk."

Many of the log cabins were 12'x20' and exceedingly small. They were easy to keep warm. But, they would drive a sane person crazy from being so confined.

Leaving the village, we climbed for an hour and enjoyed a long downhill coast on the other side. Nice to go fast again after creeping up the hill. That road continued in high gear for ten miles. Huge billowing thunderheads mushroomed into the sky behind us--pure white against a tantalizingly blue sky.

The road meandered through more wilderness as we picked up a new river and headed for Hot Sulphur Springs. We promised ourselves a half gallon of orange juice when we arrived. I guzzled down the entire half gallon within minutes. Extreme thirst on a hot day causes a gluttony unimaginable to anyone who is constantly satisfied.

We headed out of the town with a treacherous 25 mph head wind. The road cut a razor's edge line south and the wind made an invisible wall pushing north. It was an unholy butt-busting muscle job trying to push into the wind. After two hours, we reached a stack of hay in an open field. It was 6:00 p.m. and the sun neared dusk. There wasn't a tree for miles and, as usual, we stopped out in the middle of nowhere.

Some may ask what it's like pushing into a head wind. I've pushed into breezes at 10 mph and gales at 50 mph. Merciless and miserable! They grind a rider down and make for suffering that seems eternal. If there was a hell, it would be an eternal head wind. Every muscle fights the onslaught and it feels useless to go against the wind. But it's a part of bike touring and must be dealt with in a cheerful and positive manner. A smile and a good attitude make it easier. But if you want to know the real truth, head winds SUCK!

I hate them like I hate sauerkraut and liver. I hate head winds like I hate a bad case of sunburn or poison ivy. I especially hate head winds like I hate mustard and ketchup on my pancakes. Or salt in my wounds, or a headache while making love, or being run over by a Mack truck in my dreams, or George Bush being re-elected for a third term, or 20 mosquitoes in my tent...it goes on. Now that I've got that out of my system, I feel better.

We cooked dinner and since we camped near a haystack, we, as they say, hit the 'hay' and fell asleep.

Rain and lightning split the sky ahead of us in the morning. The majestic peaks in front of us vanished in the battleship gray sky that hung like a blanket across the land. Marching cloud soldiers played among the peaks. It seemed like they saw us coming and marched toward us.

At first, a few droplets fell. Then more and finally, a drizzle. The pavement took the first splats like someone dropping BB's from the sky. A rooster tail rose off Denis' back tire. We rode in the thick of rain--but we kept a steady pace--past Ringsby and on to Walsill. The sky opened up like someone draining Hoover Dam.

With not too many moments to spare, we stopped at a restaurant to eat and read for the next two hours. Outside, our bikes leaned against the glass. Condor dripped wet with dirty rims. The panniers sagged from the water weight. Beyond the eves of the building, it rained cats and dogs. Have you ever wondered where that saying came from? Who in their right mind would say it and why?

I found out from an old rancher who had driven up in a pickup truck. He was in town to buy groceries. We got into a conversation when he said, "It's been raining cats and dogs for the last week now."

"Do you have any idea where that saying came from?" I asked.

"Sure," he said. "Raining cats and dogs goes back many hundreds of years to the Dark Ages, when people believed in all sorts of ghosts, goblins and witches, and even thought that animals, like cats and dogs, had magical powers. The cat was thought by sailors to have a lot to do with storms, and the witches that were believed to ride in the storms were often pictured as black cats. Dogs and wolves were symbols of winds and the Norse storm god Odin was frequently shown surrounded by dogs and wolves. So, when a particularly violent storm came along, people would say it was raining cats and dogs....with the cat symbolizing the rain and the dogs representing the wind and storm."

"That's great," I said. "Thank you very much."

"You're welcome," he said. "I better get my stores back to the ranch or the wife won't be fixing me dinner."

"Take care," I said as he walked into the grocery.

Later, I talked with the cashier lady in the adjacent grocery store. She had been married 55 years to the same man. She talked about her kids and how proud she was of them. I asked her about her favorite accomplishments in her life. Raising five kids was her greatest adventure.

In the end, that is the most important adventure any parent can have. Good for her!

We shoved off into a moderate rainfall. Gray skies and brown, windswept prairie carried us toward distant mountains. We reached Livingston, an old railroad town, where cowboys drove pickup trucks and rode horses. A great railroad museum offered a glimpse into our not so distant past.

Denis suffered a flat on our way out of town. Later, we turned off 89 onto Route 547 and it proved the nicest stretch of quiet highway we had ridden--with mountains on our left and a wide valley on our right. The Yellowstone River flowed back north. Ranches dotted the valley and fences made for patches of land from hay crops to wheat and some corn. Horses munched grass along with cows and goats. Peace and tranquility would describe the scene we pedaled through.

However, as we headed south along the wide Yellowstone River, a black, ominous storm front moved toward us. We watched a squall line of rain pouring from the sky like a giant gray curtain being dragged over the land. It was headed toward us.

But we couldn't find a campsite with all the farms and no trespassing signs. We rode into a pine-covered creek, but there was no place to camp, so we headed into the storm hoping to find a place. No luck! The front was no more than 20 minutes before hitting us. Finally, we came upon a small triangle of land not fenced off.

"This is home for the night," I said to Denis as I wheeled Condor over the grass and leaned him up against the barbed wire fence.

"We must pitch our tents quickly," he said.

Minutes later, we pitched camp. The sheet of rain kept coming at us. We pulled the packs from the bikes and tossed them into the tents. We covered the bike seats with plastic as the first drops started. By the time we zipped up the rain flies, the sky unloaded. It slapped the tents and lightning crackled across the sky with spaghetti fingers hitting the ground. The downpour slammed us with its fury.

Nonetheless, being the neighborly type, Denis invited me over for hot soup, pasta sauce, bread and tea. He cooked them in his vestibule. I came over in the rain and we sat huddled in his nylon home--eating our dinner. We biked 75 miles in the rain, into the dry, and finally beat the new storm by getting into our tents before it hit.

I returned to my tent to the steady drumming of the rain on the nylon. I shed my riding shorts and slipped on a fresh set of underwear. My air mattress inflated and I fluffed up my backpack with clothes to give me a soft pillow. After slipping into my warm bag, I zipped it up and stared at the roof. The rain beat down in a steady play from the sky while lightning created a strobe-like lighting effect every few minutes. For a second, the tent lit up like day and darkened just as quickly. Seconds later, rumblings echoed across the sky like someone shaking a giant piece of sheet metal. Within minutes, I was, as they say, sawing logs.

Paradise Valley along the Yellowstone River is exactly as the late TV journalist Charles Kuralt reported, "One of the prettiest and grandest stretches of highway in North America." While we pedaled, the wide, wild, untamed waters of Yellowstone River churned below us. High pine-covered mountains rose to the east and west of us. Clouds filled a sensuous blue sky above us while grasses and flowers outlined the road before us. We pedaled along a grand march through nature's showcase.

Once back on Route 89 again, we entered Yankee Jim Canyon. The river became a violent white-water cataract. The valley narrowed into a steep rock-walled passage. Fallen chunks of rock lay on the road in several places. That gave us pause!

On the river, rafters paddled their way over rapids and through the wild current. We heard their laughter and cheers. We stopped at one turnout and dipped our feet into the ice cold water. Very refreshing! Further along, we passed a unique rock formation called the "DEVIL'S SLIDE." A spine of rock heaved to a vertical column that looked like a quarter mile long slide with spikes on it like the back of one of those dinosaurs from long ago. For anyone sliding down it, there was good reason to call it something the devil would dream up to make some poor sinner miserable. Still further up the canyon, eagle nests had been built on flat platforms atop telephone poles. We watched young eagles spreading their wings, getting ready to fly.

In Gardner, we washed our clothes at Jim's Laundromat. Late in the afternoon, we faced a 1,000 foot climb in four miles to Mammoth Campground. We snapped pictures at the main entrance, which was a grand sight with a rock monument that looked like we were entering a magical kingdom.

We began our climb near the Gardiner River on the 45th parallel and entered Wyoming all at the same time. A 10 percent grade greeted us with its heart pounding, lung gasping provocation. A few rocks had fallen on the road. Danger stalked us every mile. I gnashed my teeth coming up the curves--struggling to keep the bike moving forward. I cranked Condor hard in Granny gear, which for me, was a 24 tooth front chain ring on my mountain expedition bike connected to a 34 tooth low gear on my freewheel. Condor was geared like a bulldozer which meant he could climb any grade, but, of course, I must spin the crank faster. My quads tightened up with the constant blood flow needed to feed them on such an arduous climb. I strained my hands on the handlebars as I powered my body uphill.

Near the road the Gardiner River pounded its white water into a roaring cascade of rocks and pulsing current. With each crank up such a steep grade, my lungs heaved with the need for oxygen and my heart raced. My legs pressed into the road. I felt the river's power enter me. I soaked in the sun's fading light across a meadow. Colors brightened from the back lighting at that bewitching hour. I felt hot and sweaty and cooled at the same time by the cold mist coming off the water. My goal kept extending around the bend in the road that kept forever moving upward. In a moment, the sun vanished. The sky darkened. The drama at the end of the day pulled me into its inner sanctum. On that simple uphill struggle, mini-quest if you will, I became a part of nature. Not an observer, not comfortable, not at ease, not bored and not complacent. I participated in my life.

As I watched the faces of the people passing me, they sat expressionless behind glass windows of their cars--isolated, no effort, no drama, no expenditure, and no excitement.

As Denis and I rounded the last bend, the road flattened into Mammoth Campground. We eased up our efforts and shifted into higher gears. What a triumphant feeling!

We attended a campfire program hosted by a ranger who spoke of the early years in Yellowstone. Jim Bridger, mountain man extraordinaire, told tall tales of waterfalls (geysers) going up and rivers going so fast they got hot from the friction on the rocks, which caused them to steam. In the first years, poachers killed many bison, moose, elk and beavers. They were law-breakers--cunning and clever with rifles--and ready to make a buck.

I'm always mystified why there are so many men in the world who are willing to be bad or 'evil' for the sake of money or power. Unfortunately, they are at every level of society and every country. They persist from ancient times to now. They have remorse only when they get caught. Some become rich and famous like the Kennedy 'Camelot' family that bootlegged booze during the prohibition years and others went to jail like Al Capone or John Gotti who were present day crime family figures. It's unfortunate the human race develops such people. We all pay a price and so do the animals--especially all the endangered ones over in Africa that get butchered for their horns, hands or fur.

But, money gives power and power gives energy and humans like that energy. Many theologians have wrestled with the inherent evil propensities in human kind through the centuries. Some religions have a culprit, the devil, while others say it's a curse, while others know that evil is the other side of good. It's a positive/negative universe. Is money the root of all evil? Hardly! It's another manifestation of humanity's dance.

After the ranger talk, a lady and her husband stopped me at the water spigot as I washed my dishes. They had just finished dinner outside their camper van.

"Are you one of the guys who rode a bicycle up the hill?" she asked.

"Sure am!"

"Why do you do that?" she asked with a Swiss accent.

"It's fun," I said.

"But isn't it hard work to climb up long mountain roads?" she asked.

I stood there for a moment before speaking, "Gees, I don't know how to explain that," I said. "Let me put it this way....when you started up the pass in your vehicle, did you feel any anticipation?"

"No."

"Did you use your body?"

"No."

"Did you feel the tingling fresh air coming off the river along the road?"

"No."

"Did you sweat; get hungry, thirsty and tired?"

"No."

"Did you have any triumph once you got to the top of the hill?"

"What does triumph mean in this case?" she asked.

"Well, like you accomplished something."

"No, my husband just drove into this campground."

"That's the difference," I said. "What took you five minutes, took us an hour. We poured our bodies, minds and spirits into that climb. I guess it can't be understood unless you are someone who loves physical exertion."

"I like comfort," she said. "We have a nice bed in the camper and it's warm."

"That's great," I said. "You are traveling the style that is good for you."

We bantered about a few more things before I made my way back to my tent.

I couldn't help chuckling to myself about the "C" word. It's a prime word for most women. If they don't have comfort, they're not happy. A man who loves to camp, climb, hike, ski, raft and ride--better make sure his woman is warm, dry and comfortable--or he's dead meat.

Or, he's single. Take your pick!

Down the highway the following day, we swept through a series of turns into a valley--that soon began to climb, climb and climb. Many trucks and cars passed us. As I labored up that mountain, I remembered the coyotes who had howled last night--almost a caroling for us as they raised their songs to the moon. That's why they are called "song dogs" by the Indians. In between, a couple of great horned owls added their hoot-e-hoots.

The hill kept climbing until we passed Undine Falls, a small, 30 foot drop of white water. Later we passed Lava Creek which featured sparkling waters rushing over a black lava rock surface. Later we passed a flat, grassy lake bottom called "Phantom Lake." Further up the pine tree lined road with a rocky wilderness floor, we passed Calcite Springs. A group of sulfur fumaroles steamed out of the side of a mountain and into the Gardiner River. Later, we saw the remains of a petrified tree. The road snaked through the 1988 forest fire ravaged wilderness that left thousands of acres of scorched forest. Already the new pines stood six feet tall. Renewal--all that burned had sprung forth in flowers and hope. Nature, the grand chess player of creative beauty, had triumphed. That's the thing with nature; it doesn't stand still for man or beast. We all play its game in the end.

At Tower Falls, cars loaded the parking lot. On our bikes, tourists thought of us as traveling oddities. People looked at us as if we were nuts. Many stared and the look on their faces was, "How can those two crazy people ride up and down these mountain grades...and more importantly, why?" Let 'em wonder.

Tower Falls' unique name came from the skyscraper-like rock 'towers' that stood near the falls. We walked to the falls where we took pictures and talked with a group of older ladies who were curious about our travels.

From where we were, we faced a 3,200 foot climb to the top of Dunraven Pass. I figured two and one-half hours and Denis figured an even three. We began in a drizzle which gave way to overcast skies, but no rain. The road led up and up...still further up. Along the stream, through the pine forests, along an Aspen grove--still upward toward the sky we pedaled. Cool winds kept us from sweating. The road snaked ever upward along the hillsides toward the gray sky. Stroke after stroke of the pedal, we climbed. We ate, drank and pedaled. We cranked up the mountain at four miles per hour. We gained altitude from 6,000 to 7,000 to 8,000 and beyond. We labored up the flank of that mountain--with a valley on our left.

Several cars were parked with binoculars set up on tripods. One lady said, "That's a grizzly over there next to the wood line."

Everyone excitedly turned their eyes to the spot. I strained to see the magnificent beast. Down across the green grasses, across a river and along the wood line--a huge, tan shouldered, with glossy brown fur—yes, a grizzly rummaged in a dead tree stump looking for lunch. Before me, he jerked his head upward as if toying with some meal he had found. He was BIG, maybe 900 pounds of hair, tooth and claw. I watched him for several minutes. A grizzly represents one of the grand wonders of the world. John Muir said, "We are now in the mountains and they are in us, kindling enthusiasm, making every nerve quiver, filling every pore and cell of us...how glorious a conversion, so complete and wholesome it is, scarce memory enough of old bondage days left as a standpoint to view it from."

When Muir talked about bears living an eternal life, he was right. They know not that they will die nor do they expect to die. Additionally, they don't worry about death. Humans on the other hand, come into this life dumb as a bat, but fear dying for the rest of their lives. They dream up all sorts of rituals and religions that will save them from the terror of death. In the meantime, their lives have precious time wasted that could have been lived. Thankfully, I'm like a bear and don't worry myself about death. I'll simply keep living until I die. Jack London, another friend of mine said, "I will be a fiery meteor--every inch ablaze through my life, not a sleepy comfortable planet. I will live my days well and not live to prolong them."

High words for me as I jumped back astride Condor and continued upward that led out of the valley and into a burned forest with skeleton trees standing dead by the millions. Their tan bodies, devoid of bark and needles, hung on the landscape like faceless soldiers in a war against a fire that was lost. Lost? Not really. A new generation of pines shot from the forest floor in a fresh generation.

We moved through the woods as the road meandered along the side of Washburn Mountain...still moving upward. Damn! When was this climb going to end?

"I've just about had all the climbing I can take," I said to Denis.

"Oh Frosty," he said. "Keep pedaling forever and you'll get to the top."

From the backside of forever at 6:30, we reached the top with a raging storm moving in on us. Clouds mushroomed in the valley filled with dead trees. A mist soaked the air as if it was a giant steam room at the gym. Darkness crept into the wilds. We stopped to put on our rain gear and gloves. As we got on our bikes, the rain hit. Big, fat cruel raindrops hit full force with a cold wind driving them. Down the mountain we rolled. The rain increased as we dropped into deep green forests along a river. Still further from the 9,400 foot Dunraven Pass, we flew down that valley from our high perch.

"You damned crazy man," I muttered to myself. "This is miserable. I'm freezing. My glasses are fogged, nearly blinding me, my feet are soaked, my fingers feel like icicles, my butt hurts, my legs feel like rubber, I'm 52 years old, I've got a runny nose, my shoulders hurt, and I'm flying down a 9,400 foot mountain on a bicycle in a heavy rainstorm."

Even I have to pause at times wondering why I willingly do this to myself. Is it fun? Like I told that Swiss lady in the camper van, bicycle adventure means drama. It represents the stuff of life. It is the struggle, courage, tenacity, victory and fulfillment that make it spiritual, and oh, so satisfying! I love that first bird of the morning and the last chirp at night not to mention the coyotes singing their songs. How can I deny myself these pleasures of the spirit in this overly mechanized world?

Yes, Jack London, I too am a meteor--blazing happily white hot with searing excitement across the sky of my life.

But at this moment, I am pretty miserable. This sucks!

CHAPTER 9 — VOLUPTUOUSNESS OF LIVING

"Every human capacity," Socrates said, "is amplified by energy. The mind becomes brighter, healing accelerates, strength magnifies, imagination intensifies, emotional power and charisma expand. So energy can be a blessing."

Yes, I said to myself. I felt all those things.

"But life energy must flow somewhere," his voice continued. "Where internal obstructions lie, the energy burns and if it builds up beyond what an individual body or mind can tolerate, it explodes. Anger grows into rage, sorrow turns to despair, concern becomes obsession, and physical aches become agony. So energy can also be a curse. Like a river, it can bring life, but untamed it can unleash a raging flood of destruction."

"What can I do now?" I asked, talking to the air.

Memories of Socrates' wisdom echoed in my mind: "The body will do whatever it has to in order to bleed off excess energy. If it isn't spent consciously, in creative endeavors, physical activity, or sexual relations, then the subconscious will blow off this energy in fits of anger or cruelty, nightmares, crime, illness, or through abuse of alcohol, tobacco, other drugs, food or sex. Untamed energy, meeting internal obstacles, is the source of all addictions. Don't try to manage the addictions--clear the obstructions!"

Dan Millman "Sacred Journey of the Peaceful Warrior"

For an hour, through rain, cold and misery, we splashed our way down the mountain in that nasty storm. Usually, coasting down a pass is a gleeful, fun-filled, ecstatic time. It feels like being a kid enjoying a free ride. Not this one!

By the time we reached the Grand Canyon of Yellowstone, we suffered hypothermia and great hunger! We checked into the hiker-biker campsite and pitched our tents. The rain stopped, but cold numbed us. Denis and I fired up our stoves for our welcomed hot chocolate treats. That first sip of heavenly 'Swiss Miss' slipped down my throat with soothing pleasure. Next, we boiled water and tossed in noodle soup. That was the best noodle soup of my life! Each sip of hot broth melted over my taste buds and gave me a joy beyond description. For the main meal, we ate rice and broccoli dipped with bread. I savored every single grain of rice and every chewy bit of broccoli. I cut a tomato into the dinner and warmed it over the rice. I couldn't have been in more pleasure than I was sitting at that picnic table with Denis and relishing every second of glorious eating.

After dinner, it was evident that I needed a shower. I hadn't taken one in five days. At the bathroom, I found an all-you-can-use hot water shower for three bucks. My body starved for a steaming hot shower, one where the soap cleans and the water clears--not only the body but the soul, too. I paid my money and stepped into the shower room. My own stall awaited. I slipped out of my wet, salty, sweaty, dirty, soaked tights, shirt, socks, shoes and shirt. I peeled off my riding gloves and helmet. Mud and road dirt spattered my glasses. I shivered and shook.

The moment I turned on the shower, a cloud of heavenly steam rose from the curtain. I stepped in with delicious anticipation. Some moments in life are said to be higher than others where one reaches a state of perfection or indescribable energy pulsing through his body. This was one of those times.

I stepped into what I call the "voluptuousness of living." I never enjoyed a shower that gave so much meaning, so much feeling and so much power as that moment from--incredible misery to welcomed pleasure. Every drop caressed my skin with warmth. I threw my head under the nozzle for a standing immersion of utter abandonment to sensory euphoria. The soap foamed on my skin and cleaned not only my body, but it washed away my troubles. While standing there, I became aware that my legs were strong and powerful. I felt thankful for their endurance and that they carried me to great heights and never complained. I gave thanks for my arms that held me to the bike. I appreciated my eyes for the visions they allowed me to see. How blessed I was to have a body that worked well and served me on my journey. Thinking further as the shower caressed my entire skin's surface, I felt thankful for my good fortune and my ability to enjoy with awe, wonder, and gratitude--this marvelous life experience. I could not have gotten to this shower and this moment of voluptuous living without having climbed Dunraven Mountain Pass. A similar ride in Kansas would not have released the incredible emotions or appreciations. Why? Because there would not have been any struggle.

I've been asked in the past which I liked better-- riding on the flats or in the mountains. "Mountains," I always say. "They bring the greatest challenges and the greatest rewards." Yet, one man said he felt sorry for me as I climbed a mountain pass.

He may not have read Aldous Huxley's "BRAVE NEW WORLD." The protagonist was born in a test tube, and his fellow human beings lived in a bubble covered city--in the future--where everything was perfect. His perfect life offered no yin or yang. He broke through his 'perfection stupor' and escaped out of the city into the "forbidden zone," which was the wilderness where he had to hunt for food and had to protect himself from insects and animals. His life became his own. He became vulnerable to normal life consequences. The "savage" said he wanted to know love, hurt, pain, joy, hunger, heat and cold.

That book changed my life. I decided I didn't want to be so comfortable that living became too easy. I didn't want to go from my air conditioned house to my climate controlled car to an office complex where everyone wore the same suits and thought the same way as they clawed their way up the corporate ladder with accompanying stress levels and ulcers, and kids going crazy because their parents were not home to guide them. Too much ease and comfort kills the spirit. I wanted to know the differences--because in the opposites, came perspective and appreciation.

I have rarely been a spectator. The result of my decision becomes more precious with each passing year as I head into the last third of my time on earth. Life sweeps along swiftly enough without spending hours and days on useless inactivity such as television. I swear the TV has become a world drug and its addiction—crippling to humanity. It's such a waste of time and life. I've figured out many answers to life's problems while riding my bike.

I've embraced life's ups and downs. I don't put myself at risk, but neither do I want to become bored or work at a job that doesn't enrich me. In that mode, life would pass by mundanely. In a twinkling, I would be on my deathbed wondering where it all went so fast. We have 70 odd years to fill up our lives, and I want to fill them with the voluptuousness of living. That, particularly! It is being aware of pain, joy and potential within myself--of being excited by every leaf on a tree as it flutters in the wind, or watching a hawk rip down from the sky to grab a mouse, or the delight of discovering a lady bug on my legs in early spring, or gazing upon a mountain as it pierces the clouds. It leads me to a kind of rage too, which is the blood sister of love--because the people of this world make it a charming, insane, exciting and confusing place. I want to maintain the ability to deal with them, with my mind, and spirit--at full bore. To see is to know and to know is to fall in love with what is known.

The hot water ran out. The cold water shocked my skin. I jumped out of the stall. I dried off and headed back to camp. I still pondered as I made my way through the darkness to our hiker-biker site.

Perhaps, as I looked around, our country enjoys too much comfort, and, like a drug, we keep moving to a higher scale of comfort and ease. When that level of comfort no longer suffices, we try for more. All the while we draw ourselves further away from vibrant living or meaningful struggle, because comfort may be, like Millman says, "an obstacle." Look at the figures of one million prescriptions of Prozac a week in this country, or the fact that Jenny Craig and Weight Watchers enjoy greater incomes than many countries' Gross National Products. Some estimate over 15 million alcoholics in the USA. Fifty million Americans smoke--resulting in nearly a half million premature deaths each year.

Excedrin and Aleve sales reach into the billions annually. Suicide is the number one killer of teenagers.

Stress clutches almost every city dweller in its grasp. Are these a result of too much comfort? Maybe it's crowding. I wish I knew because I can only speculate.

I thought of John Brown and his struggle. I sent him prayers of energy to win his battle. I thanked my lucky stars to have Denis share this grand adventure with me. I stood there thankful for a positive spirit, strong body and healthy mind. Darkness descended when I returned to camp.

"Salute Frosty," Denis said.

"Salute Denis," I said as I headed for the tent.

"Bon nuit," he said.

"Bon nuit," I said as I unzipped the screen and crawled into my tent.

We broke camp under a sunny sky the next morning and headed for Inspiration Point. For those who have never been to Yellowstone, Inspiration Point stands on the side of an awesome canyon that defies imagination. Bright tan and yellow treacherous canyon walls cut a 1,000 foot 'V' wedge through the forest. It looks like the result of a giant back-hoe from some alien civilization that dug a long ditch out of the wilderness to drain the discharge from their warp drive engines and simply left it there when they flew back into space. Both sides were lined with trees, but once the 'V' wedge of tan rock dropped downward, there was nothing but rock. Below, the raging white and emerald water of the Yellowstone River cut a crooked path a thousand feet below the point.

Ravens flew over the canyon on the updrafts created by the thermals. Above us, a brilliant blue sky, but in front of us, a grand cascading waterfall that had turned snow white as it dropped over the edge of lower falls.

We walked closer to the roaring cataract. We saw the upper falls and soon, we stood high above the lower falls. A 20 minute walk through the woods down a series of switch backs brought us to the falls themselves.

There, under a blue sky, a foot deep layer of green water poured into the canyon from the Upper Falls and raced over a flat rock bed. It made its way through a 50 foot wide opening to begin its white rage over a 300 foot vertical drop. We stood at the edge, watching. The green water turned to white. Millions of rain drops exploded out of the churning, plummeting water and were blown by the wind as if they were a covey of pigeons circling in the air. In the main body of the descending torrent, huge explosions of water blasted outward as if someone had set dynamite charges inside the cliff. We surmised that the water bounced off jutting rocks in the cliff wall, causing the water to explode outward. Below, an all white cloud erupted where the water hit bottom.

So much mist rose from the base that a dozen instant waterfalls cascaded down the sides of the sandstone cliffs. Everywhere, the mist blew, green plants grew on the cliff faces. From the peaceful view at Inspiration Point, we enjoyed nature's power creating a wild, foaming, roaring, raging, deafening, unbridled force of water before us. The misty air filled our lungs with energy.

A full double rainbow reflected off the mist that formed from the raging water dropping over the falls. Each time the water shifted, the mist created new waterfalls that raged down the yellow and gold sandstone. Bright green moss covered the rocks near the falls, but gave way to tan rock away from the waters. What made the scene so eye popping were the colors and rock cliffs in blazing red and yellow mixed into a mosaic like

Grandma's multicolored quilt. But all eyes focused on the forever white water raging over the massive precipice. Walking onto the gargantuan scene for the first time etched a picture of nature's grace--a simple serenity that moves through the eyes and settles into one's heart and creates a place of peace in the spirit.

Back at the top, we mounted our bikes. We headed toward Norris Geyser twelve miles away. As I pedaled, I knew that energy from the falls was one more source of power for me to enjoy in my memory.

The road led up and down through burned trunks of trees from the 1988 fire. A coyote crossed our path and looked at us with indifference as he ducked into the woods and trotted about his daily business.

At Norris Geyser, an entire lake bed filled with blue water and steaming vents—startled our senses. Boardwalks carried people to closer views of the boiling ponds.

Again on the bikes, we pedaled from 8,000 feet to 7,000 to 6,000 feet along the Gibbon River. We pedaled effortlessly to rest our legs after the ordeal of yesterday where we climbed half way to heaven but it felt like hell on our bodies. And, when we reached the top, it was not the Pearly Gates and angels in wings, but cold rain and misery.

Along Gibbon River, we passed through Elk Meadow where a dozen elk grazed beside the river. Hawks above and elk below. Blue sky, green pine and sparkling rivers! Two dozen cars full of people shot pictures of the animals. If we had been there in mid summer, it would have been a crowded nightmare. We made our way along the river which entered a steep canyon. The river turned to silver with the sun ahead of us. Many times it roared into white water. At one point, it cascaded into a bridal veil at Gibbon Falls.

The 14 miles to Madison campground gave us more sightseeing because we pedaled effortlessly with a three percent downhill grade. We rode in a gleeful 'zone' while pedaling and stopping to smell the flowers along the way. We stopped at Beryl Springs with a boiling water source that created a steaming caldron. However, it made our noses want to crawl inside our faces because of its steamy rotten egg smell.

Although we camped at Madison, we called it "Camp Motor Home" because there wasn't a tent in the whole place. One hundred motor homes filled the campground. They featured all shapes and sizes, mostly 35 to 45 feet long and towing cars. They equaled the size of a Greyhound bus. Many had satellite dishes blooming like hibiscus flowers from their roofs so they could watch the latest important episode of Jerry Springer. The motor homes featured hydraulic jacks that leveled the vehicle automatically. They featured generators, electrics and sewage hookups.   Inside--refrigerators, microwaves, four burner gas stoves, air conditioning, dishwashers, showers, electric blankets, stereo, video and heated toilet seats. Now that's what I call getting back to nature and roughing it.

I walked to the camp bathroom, which featured hot and cold running water, baby wipes, baby changing table in the men's side (we've lost it men), flush toilets, and even paper covers for the toilet seats. Paper towels and blow dryers were added along with mirrors on the wall with soap dispensers. The place proved as spotless as a hospital operating room. A heater came on whenever the temperature dropped outside to make that restroom a palace. More roughing it!

Whatever happened to the old outhouse? I used to carry my roll of TP, and approach it with caution, especially if it was down wind. I unlatched the door, took a deep breath and entered the dark, wood confines. Light slipped through a half moon cut into the door. Upon entering, spiders fled across their webs and I elbowed the cob webs off to the side. A square wood door flap covered the round hole on a bench. Sometimes a ragged Sears catalog lay beside the hole. Rays of light filtered through the cracks. By the time I sat down, I exhaled my lung full of air and sucked in through my shirt to filter the deadly poisonous air blowing out of the bowels of the pit like a demon trying to kill me.   Hoping to do my business as quickly as possible, I exhaled again and breathed in little bits of air, trying not to knock myself out with the deadly gas.

At the same time, I inspected the hole for spiders as I hated spiders crawling across my rear-end or dangling from my most precious possessions. Nothing worse than a spider spinning a web from me to the lower insides of the outhouse.   I couldn't imagine what they snared down in those dark depths. When I was a kid on the farm, I used to think there was a monster of the muck and that he might drag me down into the darkness.

Quickly seating myself, I did my business, pulled up my pants, grabbed the roll of TP, tucked in my shirt and took one last gasp of air so as not to pass out from lack of oxygen and made my way out of the outhouse with as much dignity as possible. Oh, the thrill of it all! One never lives such an experience in this modern age. Such a pity!

That night, it hit 25 degrees and I felt it as I curled deeper into my bag and zipped the hood around my head. It's a special comfort sleeping on an air mattress night after night inside a mummy bag--confined and limited--yet warm and cozy.

After we ate breakfast, the road climbed up a long hill but leveled and dropped along the Fire Hole River. It shimmered in the morning sun. Although shallow, it flowed fast over its rock bed.

We rode along steaming thermal pools, burned wilderness everywhere, and, a moose. Yes, a young, horned moose! I took a couple of shots. He munched grass in the woods. We passed a few geysers until we came to the Fountain Paint Pot geyser area. Several pools boiled and steamed 100 feet into the crisp morning air. We heard and saw a wild fumerole that sounded like an air compressor. Another pond featured beige-colored mud that bubbled and splattered at the surface. Another pot boiled up clear turquoise water.

Standing there, it was amazing to me that this earth still has a molten liquid core that reaches to the surface once in a while to blow off excess lava like Mount Saint Helens in 1980. Deep inside this planet, liquid rock still rages billions of years after the earth was born. How can it keep those temperatures hot enough to keep the rock liquid? It seems like it must have some kind of energy reactions or nuclear fission like the sun. Otherwise, it would have cooled off by convection of the oceans sucking heat away from it in the last six billion years or so of this planet's existence. For most of us on this earth, it will be a continuing intellectual discussion, or simply ignored because it's for the scientific minds to figure out. Even if they do, it's still goes about its business.

Denis and I stood where Jim Bridger had stood. We saw what he saw, but we saw it 200 years later. Still the same activity! I felt humbled to travel to this place in the universe where the wonders of nature startle the senses and excite the imagination.

Finally we reached Old Faithful--the granddaddy of all geysers. The parking lot, even in September, filled with cars for the hourly spectacle. We watched a movie in the theater and stopped outside to see Old Faithful explode into the air. It rose slowly as the water followed up through the steam and climbed to 150 feet, held it for a few seconds and dropped back down to a steaming vent. Around us, a dozen other lesser geysers steamed in all corners of the area. People walked on boardwalks with kids and grand parents.

Again on our bikes, we pedaled over 8,200 foot Craig Pass and swooped down again, only to climb over Norris Pass at 8,300 feet--which carried us over the Continental Divide twice. That second downhill took us down to the huge 136 square mile Yellowstone Lake. It reflected dark blue with pines surrounding it.

Our day filled with rivers, canyons, geysers, moose, elk, deer, coyote, buffaloes, and hawks.

We pitched camp at a hiker-biker and proceeded to eat everything in sight. We enjoyed great anticipation of the evening meal. Stark raving starvation was more like it. Denis cooked pasta with a big jar of tomato sauce.

"This is the greatest meal you have ever cooked," I said to Denis.

He smiled, "You devour everything in sight, mon ami."

As we sat there, the sun created a pink glow across the sky while it descended into the trees. The air cooled which made the food taste even better. All around us, lodge pole pines struck tall profiles against the evening sky. The last chirps of the birds created a soft ending to the day. Cheep, cheep, crackle, crackle, warble, warble-- and the abrupt base sound of a raven.

The steaming pot of pasta cooked to perfection. We scooped it into our pans and shoveled the warm food into our mouths. We added a bit of bread with each mouthful.

Sitting there, a black canopy of stars hung over our heads. On a bicycle adventure, I look up often at the night sky and thank my lucky stars to be alive.

It was a most voluptuous moment.

CHAPTER 10 — EMERGING CREATIVE ENERGY

"There is more to life than increasing its speed."

Gandhi

Sometime in the night, it started raining--small drops at first and soon--a deluge. It rained the rest of the night and into the morning.

When I unzipped the tent, marvelously clean air burst into my lungs. Not a single particulate or puff of car exhaust was in it—just fresh, clean air. Sure beats breathing in a city.

I know that living in the Denver area, I breathe that brown cloud full of toxins day and night, every minute of the year. I tolerate it, but my body suffers from it.

Before we hit the road, the rain began.

"Darn! I figured if it rained all night," I said to Denis. "It wouldn't rain all the next day."

"Better look to the sky again," Denis said.

In front of us, a black, ominous cloud boiled low in the heavens. The sky behind it burst with water. We stopped at the ranger station to put on our rain gear. The ironic aspect about bicycling rain gear is that I may stay dry from the rain, but get wet from the sweat. Either way, I'm soaked.

Before we reached the highway, an earnest rain fell upon us. We cranked south knowing we would soon be soaking wet. Since it had rained all night, the air felt uncommonly clean and energized with moisture. Our lungs filled with energy.

However, mile after mile, the rain began its onslaught upon our mutual misery. We looked like a couple of mongrel dogs that ran through a drainage ditch. Cars splashed us on the down hills. My glasses fogged.

While pedaling, it reminded me of the daily hot rain I suffered in the Brazilian rain forest in the interior of South America. Big fat raindrops splatted against my helmet and jacket--and all around me grew lush, green jungle--steaming as it soaked up the water. Rain soaked me from head to toe. But even with the rain and the mildewed packs, I lived a unique adventure. I rode far away from home and far away from comfort--yet I was at home in the world. How many people are so blessed to cycle the length of South America? I had put myself there, so I accepted it.

"I'm so wet, I've finally become a 185 pound raindrop," I said to Denis when we stopped for a snack.

"Make those two raindrops," he said.

"I wonder how John is doing today," I said to Denis from out of the blue.

"I think of him often as we pedal down the road," Denis said. "He is a good man with a big heart. He will win his battle against cancer. I am sure of it."

We both nodded that John Brown's battle made our rainstorm struggle miniscule by comparison.

We cruised along Lake Lewis and then along the Lewis River where it dropped into deep canyon white water below us. All around, the new green pines from the 1988 burn grew skyward. They gave promise as they poked their green needles upward among the burned out telephone pole skeletons from the fires. In 50 years, the forest would be totally renewed. That meant a mere blink in geologic time.

We cruised through four hours of rain. As we passed out of Yellowstone, the guards took one look and felt so sorry for us; they let us pass by without seeing our tickets. Rain kept falling as we moved southward.

After climbing a long hill, we coasted to Jackson's Lake with a glimpse of the Grand Tetons. Named by a romantic French explorer who thought he had seen the finest breasts nature had ever created, the term Grand Tetons means "large breasts." They were, indeed, spectacular in their grandeur.

However, nothing in a Victoria Secret catalog could hold those babies! Cross Your Heart or Maiden Form? Forget it!

"Viva La Grand Teton!" I yelled out with abandon.

"Frosty," Denis yelled. "Calm down. What are you so excited about?"

"Sorry Denis," I said. "I forget myself in the moment."

We made our way along the lake shore until we reached the visitor's center. There we saw "Return of the Bison" and "The Fate of the Grizzly." Both films gave us an excellent view of wilderness management.

After the movie, it started to rain, but for a brief pause, the sun shined over the Tetons and formed a brilliant rainbow in the trees to the east. It blazed across the sky with the top of the colors in red, yellow, blue and purple.

As I sit here on this picnic table in the hiker-biker section, I'm aware of the constant presence of pine trees growing overhead. They remain eternally quiet and only whisper when the wind blows through them.

Tonight, they remain silent, but already, a pack of coyotes yelps somewhere in the distance. A gray camp robber flies above me waiting for a hand out. His buddy, a Stellar Blue Jay plays coy in the branches above me, because he too, wants a piece of bread. A short distance away, a squirrel chatters his machine gun jabber through the woods. Trees make this world possible. Strong trunks thrust out of the ground to reach for the sky. Their limbs branch outward to catch the light.

Each needle, however, holds a drop of crystal clear rain. Those drops glisten through the green. They fall from the brown cones and hit the ground. I am very aware of being within the element of nature as I hear the rain splashing about me. I move to my tent as rain drops splash on the nylon. It's rhythmic and peaceful. The trees stand as sentinels in this thriving quietness.

Later, Denis prepares a hot dinner and I'm sipping my steaming chocolate. We're just 'out here' in the wilds. I swear, it's a drug and I'm higher than a kite right now. It doesn't get any better than this.

In the morning, we headed into a cloud-covered sky. Gray mist socked in the mountains. Huge, tumbling gray clouds hugged the flanks of the Grand Tetons. But over our heads, the sky held its water for most of the day.

Along the route, the Tetons opened up every once in awhile, offering us magnificent views of jagged peaks and ice floes. Mount Moran featured five glaciers. Eight miles south, we reached Oxbow Bend where I anticipated hundreds of migrating birds in the shallows of the Snake River. Several years previously, I had seen 500 to 1,000 birds of several species cruising in the still waters of the bend. The massive and graceful white pelicans with black tipped wings resembled float planes. They glided along the river with exceptional grace and style.

But today, they were not there. A few ducks paddled leisurely on the waters.

However, we met Hans and his wife Erika from Germany. They visited the states for some scientific conferences, but found time for some sightseeing. We struck up a conversation about bikes and traveling. Hans had been a bike racer back home so he was more than a little interested in our bicycle touring. I could tell his spirit was remembering the times he was on his bike and how he would like to be on a bike again. Once a cyclist, always a cyclist! It's something that sneaks into your blood, heart and mind. It's that smooth, even flow through the air and the rhythm of pedaling that makes a person's heart beat faster. The passion rises. My bet is that when Erika and he returned home, they jumped on their bikes and pedaled around for the day! It was so nice to meet them and their enthusiasm attracted us.

After talking for awhile, we took some pictures and headed south. As we waved goodbye, I couldn't help smiling that I had made some new friends. E-mail magic makes long distance friendship quite easy with the click of a mouse. In 1989, I met Reinhold and Monika, also from Germany and we have become great friends. They visited me for our 10th anniversary of our meeting this past summer. We had such a grand time hiking and enjoying dinner-theater in Colorado.

The road we followed would take us under the nose of the jagged Teton peaks.

While we pedaled along, I shared with Denis some of my friends' crazy choices in life and the consequences they had experienced or were experiencing. I told him about my crazy choices and what they had cost me. He absorbed all my words and returned with, "There are no rules to be happy," he said. "Each of us takes a certain path and sometimes we succeed and often we fail."

I had to chuckle, because it was true. There are no rules to happiness.

We traveled along a rolling highway that flattened as it neared the lake and passed under the imposing glaciers and massive gray rock of the 13,000 foot Tetons. We resembled ants making our way past the throne room of the mountain gods. The peaks popped into and out of the clouds giving us spectacular views. The Tetons rose as jagged, raw and powerful as any mountains in the USA. They looked like shark's teeth ripping into the sky, and, at the top, aspirin-white snow filled deep canyons of gray rock. The whole line of the Tetons offers one of the most rugged on this continent.

While heading south under a tentative sky, we met a Kiwi couple and a Japanese rider moving north. We stopped and talked awhile. They were headed across the USA to Virginia--dropping south as the winter moved in.

Still further down the road, we cruised along a smooth highway all the way into Jackson where we ate at an all-you-can-eat Pizza Hut.

Denis sat in the saddle at the bar of the Million Dollar Cowboy Saloon. The place was famous for its gnarled wood, saddles instead of seats, silver dollars covering the bar and country music. Clint Eastwood made a movie in Jackson that had to do with bare knuckle fighting.

Near town, we stopped at a bird sanctuary to see a hundred ducks 'ducking' for food in the waters of the Snake River. We camped by the river.

In the morning, a hundred Canada geese took off into a low-hanging cloud. What a fabulous sight watching them form into chevrons of 20 or more and slicing through the sky with exquisite grace! It sounded like a bunch of fog horns repeating themselves across the sky. Two trumpeter swans paddled around the waters with their special grace. As the sun rose over the mountains, they too, took to the sky. Out in the cattails, hundreds of blackbirds flew in a large group as if they were a flying ameba. The 'emerging form' changed shape and shifted as the group flew indolently around the tops of the grasses--finally landing in mass in the cattails again.

I've been amazed all my life as to how those flocks of birds fly without crashing into each other. Recently, I found out why. Scientists studying flocks of birds with high-speed film made a remarkable discovery. They found that birds react faster to subtle movements of the flock than they do to signals from their own brains. As the flock veers to avoid a predator, or is moving through the sky in search of food, each bird takes about 1/70th of a second to mirror a neighboring bird's change of direction. That is less than the reaction time of an individual bird. The flock veers, swoops, and changes shape like a living thing, gracefully evading a predator and each other. Yet, no intelligence guides it. It's driven solely by the mindless reaction of each bird to the movements of its neighbor. It's called the "Swarm Factor."

Standing there, I watched that swarm moving over the reeds along the river.

We pulled out of Jackson riding beside the Snake River. The canyon narrowed for 13 miles as we rode up and down, up and down like being on the back of a roller coaster until we turned south on 191. Snow had fallen in the high country above 12,000 feet. It was cold, but we kept warm via our constant pedaling. A new river, the Hoebeck, followed along with us. On both sides, the mountains became our gateway to warmer weather. The sky turned crystal clear with Pillsbury Doughboy clouds floating in groups across the peaks.

Three hours later, we climbed out of the valley. At the top, the prairie dominated with sagebrush growing everywhere, and pronghorn antelope grazing off to the side. No trees. The road swept before us through rolling hills--and, we discovered a tailwind with a two percent downhill grade. We shifted into our highest gears and pedaled effortlessly. From our usual 12 mph, our speed jumped to 23. For the next half-hour, we 'flew' in the 'zone' of bicycling heaven where we were like two eagles soaring over the earth at low altitude. Our pedals kept rotating over the pavement, softly feathering--about to touch down--but rose again. The spokes glistened in the sun and the chains kept a steady tension of power to the rear wheels. We floated along as if two unfettered souls, flawlessly free of limits.

That 'satori' overwhelmed our senses and we hit the sweet spot in cycling where light, air, metal, rubber and body become one. It lasted for a half-hour of ecstasy.

We remembered that day for the purity of the cycling experience.

Nearing Pinedale, three billboards caught our attention. Out in the middle of nowhere, they spoke volumes to passing motorists. One worked on the famous Marlboro Country theme: Two men rode ponies into one of those romanticized western sunsets when the first man said, "Bill, I have emphysema."

The second one followed a few miles down the road with two guys branding a steer by a fire inside a corral, "Bob, I miss my lung."

The third showed a camel in bed, "I thought they called you Joe Camel."

"Change that to Joe Cardiac," the camel said.

The first one made us laugh and the second one saw us grinning. It was interesting to watch the struggle going on in the USA with tobacco folks promoting their deadly product in smoke and chew--while the health side tried to encourage all kids to not start smoking. Yet, 3,000 teens start smoking every day in America.

On the alcohol front, merchants use every advertising trick in the book to promote drinking and yet 22,000 automobile deaths each year are directly related to drunk drivers. With domestic abuse in the millions and related to alcohol, the human toll of beer and liquor is not a pretty picture that represents the country.

In the end, everyone picks their pathway, or as Millman says, "…deals with their obstructions." We remain a capricious species and subject to the whims of our ever active minds. This life journey allows us many choices in a free country. Not all choices are wise and many get us or others killed. It's all the luck of the draw or the spin of the wheel.

After the billboards, we passed a few houses where junk piled up in the yards. Some were abandoned. It causes me dismay that because of private property rights, millions of human slobs legally trash the country with wrecked cars, piles of trash, old farm implements and endless assortments of junk. It's ugly, scars the land, and shows pathetic disregard for the earth's beauty--and it's legal.

At the campgrounds in Pinedale, we met a Swiss couple riding for six months in North America. They were honeymooning and deliriously and deliciously in love. Nice to see such passion and they were well suited for each other. I tried to interest them in the mountain man exhibit in town, but they weren't into it.

That night, it dropped down to 10 degrees and I froze my butt off because my bag was only good to 20 degrees. I shivered most of the night. I was so cold; it reminded me of the year before when I worked in Antarctica and took a ride on my bicycle after a howling storm. In the morning, a whiteout howled across McMurdo Station, Antarctica with 100 mile per hour winds and minus 80 degree temperatures. I had been confined to my barracks for two days as a 'Condition One' storm worked its way over the ice pack.

By late evening, the weather turned placid but a biting 30 degrees below zero temperature kept most people inside. I, however, bundled into my cold weather gear and headed out the door to ride my bicycle onto the ice runway. Yes, there were bicycles at the scientific station for me to ride. There was a report of some emperor penguins on the ice. I must see them no matter what the cold. (Yes, I'm aware that you dear reader have now judged me to be completely out of my mind) I jumped on the bike looking like an overstuffed bear wearing all my cold weather gear. My breath vaporized as I rode toward the ice covered ocean. My lungs burned with each inhalation of polar cold. About 300 meters across the way, the setting sun glinted off the roof of Robert Falcon Scott's Hut. He had died 80 years ago on his last attempt to reach the South Pole. The Hut stood on the point of McMurdo Sound since 1902. It gave mute testimony to the courage those men displayed in their polar adventures. This was a cold, miserable place.

I rode along a path that led toward the ice pack in the sound. It's hard to describe pack-ice, but it's jumbled-broken ice chards being heaved and smashed into multiple shapes; triangles, domes, squares, tubulars and wedges--like an erector set gone crazy. However, near the shore, it was reasonably smooth with a thin veneer of snow from the blizzard.

Above me, a gold and purple sky glowed brazenly in its final glory into the crevasses of the Royal Society Range across the sound. For once, a rare quiet softened the bitter edge of the crystal white desert before me. One of the glaciers, more than ten miles across at its terminus, radiated liquid gold from the setting sun. Riding over the ice, my wheels crunched into the pack, but the fat mountain tires held their own. Even with the polar weather gear protecting my body, the numbing cold crept through the air, as if it were trying to find a way into my being.

The bike frame creaked at the cold and the tires made a popping sound on the snow I pedaled over. The big boots I wore made it hard to keep on the pedals. But I persevered and kept moving forward.

Across the ice, I looked through the sunlight and saw four black figures approaching. I shaded my eyes with my gloved hand. They drew closer, their bodies back lit by the sun on the horizon. It was a family of Emperor penguins. I dismounted from my bike. From our survival classes, I learned to sit down so as not to frighten them. By appearing smaller than them, they might find me interesting.

Slowly, I lowered myself into the snow, cross-legged, like an Indian chief. Minute by minute, they waddled closer--straight toward me. Three big birds, about 80 pounds each, kept moving dead-on in my direction. The smallest followed behind them.

Another minute passed and they were within 30 feet of me. The lead Emperor carried himself like a king. His silky black head-color swept to the back of his body and through his tail. A bright crayon yellow and orange streaked along his beak like a Nike logo 'swoosh.' Under his cheek, soft aspirin-white feathers poured downward, glistening with lanolin. His wings were black on the outside and mixed with black and white on the front. He stood at least 40 inches tall and his enormous three-toed feet were a gray reptilian roughness with blunted talons sticking out. He rolled his head, looking at me in a cockeyed fashion, as if I was the strangest creature he had ever seen.

I don't know what made me do it, but I slipped my right hand out of my glove and moved it toward him--slowly. The rest of the penguins closed in. The big guy stuck his beak across the palm of my hand and twisted his head, as if to scratch himself against my skin. I felt glossy feathers against my hand. He uttered a muffled coo. The rest of the penguins cooed. Their mucus membranes slid like liquid soap over their eyes every few seconds. I stared back, wanting to say something to them, but realized I could not speak their language. However, at that moment, we shared a consciousness of living.

My frozen breath vapors hung in the air briefly before descending as crystals toward the ground. I battled to keep from bursting with excitement. Within seconds, one of the other penguins pecked my new friend on the rump. He drew back. With that he turned and waddled away.

Following the elders, the little one gave one last look at me, as if he too wanted to scratch my hand, but was afraid, and turned with his friends. As they retreated, their wings spread out, away from their bodies like children trying to catch the wind in their arms. The baby Emperor was the last to go.

My hand turned numb so I stuck it back into the glove. As I sat there, I remembered once when a hummingbird landed on my finger--and I remembered the sheer delicacy nature shared with me that warm spring day in the Rocky Mountains. There, in that frozen wasteland beyond the borders of my imagination where man does not belong, nature touched me again with its pulsing heart and living warmth. I only hope my species learns as much respect for our fellow travelers as they show toward us.

I stood up, tightened the hood and looked for the penguins. They were gone. Only the pack ice rumbled toward the horizon. I turned to my bike. It's hard to believe that two rubber tires laced together with spokes and rims--and attached to a metal frame could carry me from the Amazon jungles, to Death Valley and on to where the bolt goes into the bottom of the globe. That simple machine lying in the frozen snow had taken me to far flung places on this planet and it had allowed me magical moments beyond description. That moment with the penguins was probably the best it had ever done by me. I remounted it and turned toward the barracks. The ride back didn't seem so cold.

But the reality was, I froze my butt off by the time I got back.

CHAPTER 11 — DARING ADVENTURE

"What a joy it is to feel the soft, spring earth under my feet once more, to follow grassy roads that lead to ferny brooks where I can bathe my fingers in a cataract of rippling notes, or to clamber over a stone wall into green fields that tumble and role and climb in riotous gladness! For me, life is either a daring adventure, or it is nothing. Security is mostly superstition. It does not exist in nature."

Helen Keller

Denis and I shook off the ice from our tents and waited for the sun to melt the remaining crystals from the nylon. We experienced the coldest night of the trip. After a hot oatmeal breakfast, we headed to the Mountain Man exhibit on the south end of town. Like the Lewis and Clark exhibit, it exceeded our expectations. Inside the museum, a movie chronicled the extraordinary saga of hundreds of men from 1824 through 1840 who moved west to trap beavers which were the rage of the fashion world from New York to London. Jim Bridger, the most famous, along with hundreds of foolhardy men--braved Indians, starvation, grizzly bears, freezing winters, disease and loneliness--just plain misery--to gain money and adventure.

They held sixteen annual rendezvous in the Pinedale area where hundreds of men and Indians came together to trade and barter. But soon, booze came into the picture and they turned out to be drunken orgies on the plains. Bridger became the only mountain man still living from the original 1824 rendezvous. The rest had been killed and others, just as foolhardy, took their places in hopes of high adventure. They got it too--arrows through their backs, legs and bellies, grizzlies munching on them for breakfast, mountain lions stalking them when their pants were down, and wolves eating their rations and attacking their horses. They starved, got deathly ill, didn't make a dime, wasted their youth and lost their lives.

Emerson said it best, "Youth, it's wasted on the young."

Being a mountain man was something I would have tried!

The museum featured stuffed animal heads on the walls. The white man slaughtered the buffalo, mountain lion, coyote, pronghorn, eagle, hawk, marmot, mountain sheep, mountain goats, and, well, just about anything he could set his rifle sights on. Mountain men trapped beaver nearly into extinction. They showcased Bridger's 49 1/2 inch flint lock rifle. The exhibit featured men who carved their name into Western lore. It reminded me of the movie Robert Redford filmed 30 years ago titled: "Jeremiah Johnson."

We may celebrate those men today, but they lived harsh lives with not much to romanticize about. They lived what they lived in their time and circumstances.

From Pinedale, we pulled into the wind and a vast prairie of rolling terrain, brilliant sky in every direction and antelope grazing peacefully in the distance. Once again, we rode out in the middle of nowhere. The asphalt road, that cut south like a knife through a baked potato, gave the only indication of human presence.

Being out in the middle of nowhere has its special flavor. When I think of my rushed, busy and pushed life back in Denver, I'm amazed if not dumbfounded to be out in a place of tumbleweed, rolling hills, wind and sky. It swallows a person in its vastness and eternalness. The winds come and go as well as the animals, and it doesn't mean anything to the land. Looking further into the landscape, I realized how tiny I was in the expanse of the universe.

I'm amazed how different men in government, or movie and sports stars seem to think of themselves as so huge, so big, so important—when in fact, they are no different than a stallion or bull fighting for the prize of the top turf or the most attractive female. One of Denver's baseball players said he wouldn't stay with the Rockies last spring if he wasn't appreciated enough. So, management paid $70 million to keep him 'loyal' to Denver fans. The management boasted the money proved an investment in the future for the club. All it did was raise the ticket prices for all those fans that have nothing better to do on a Saturday than watch someone else play a game. I'd rather be playing my own sand-lot game than watch a bunch of hotshots play for more money in one season than most people make in a lifetime. Even if they won the pennant for Denver, it wouldn't change anyone's life whatsoever. But for the guy who got the $70 million, he's laughing his butt off. At the money he's making, let's hope he feels appreciated.

Nonetheless, no matter how much money or how famous they become, those sports stars or politicians, in reality, are so unimportant to the universe.

As I pedaled through that vast nothingness of tumbleweed and wind, I accepted that I was another organism spending my allotted time as I chose--making my existence meaningful to me. Yet, I knew that in the end, it didn't mean anything except to me, and only while I was alive. This great living adventure allows us precious little time. Yogi Berra said, "It ain't over till it's over." But when it is, I will no longer be breathing to worry about it.

As we sat in the campsite in Farsom, which happened to be a green little city park with picnic tables, a ragged looking man with a pony tail rode in on a mountain bike with little in his panniers and gear. He sported big 2.25 tires which were meant for riding in dirt. He looked powerful with a wiry frame. He showed a wild look. He also smiled like a man who was happy with the world.

"Ride far today?" I asked.

"From Jackson," he said.

"Jackson!" I said. "That's 140 miles back."

"About 137 to be exact," he said.

"You've got a pair of strong legs, mate," I said.

Charlie had been cycling the Continental Divide but had been riding all the dirt trails alone. He was a former chiropractor in California, but after getting sick of people complaining to him all day long about being sick, he took up farming in Oregon. After harvesting and before planting season, he took extended rides around the country. He was pretty funny and upbeat. We talked biking until we were too tired to talk.

Leaving Farsom, the three of us pedaled over prairie grasslands, seemingly in the middle of nowhere, going nowhere. We traded places in line all day as we headed south toward Rock Springs. Charlie enjoyed riding with us just for the company and a chance to share some talking time. He turned out to be a likeable guy.

I'll never forget how he described he would rather throw a wrench at a piece of farm machinery than deal with a patient with a bad back. He said most people don't care about their health until they lose it. That's when they want a magic bullet to cure them. That's why the drug industry makes obscene profits.

We continued along with sagebrush rolling across the road and a sky that looked like the color of faded 1950s blue bathroom tile. It wasn't dramatic, but it wasn't gray. I couldn't imagine being on a horse and making only 20 miles per day. Today, we have no idea of the hardships and difficulties it took to explore that vast western region. However, I must admit that my brother Howard rode his horse, Misty, coast-to-coast across America. From Savannah, Georgia to Newport Beach, Oregon, Howard endured six months and 3,100 miles of grinding horseback riding on his epic quest to ride a horse across America.

The ride into Rock Springs presented a 1,000 foot descent off the high plateau into a town that earned its name because it was a land of rocks, rocky butts and more rocks.

Charlie rented a KOA campsite, so we decided to pile in on him. I took a 45 minute shower. Heavenly!

Up with the sun. We couldn't help it as I-80 featured roaring diesels along the highway all night. Even with my earplugs, I heard their din through my sleep. We hit the ground running at dawn to see the sun peaking over the Wyoming horizon. A full silver sky gave us a thin crescent moon and the North Star still shone above us.

We bid farewell to Charlie, Stephen and Christine. They headed along the western route through the Flaming Gorge. That meant they had to ride 12 miles into a 20 mph head wind. We never saw them again.

We pushed south and by 10:00 a.m., we had climbed 500 feet and kept climbing. We pedaled through rolling hills that turned into flat-topped mountains. By 11:00, head winds buffeted us with brutish force.

The road ribboned southward in front of us as it dipped along the vacant nothingness of the gorge. On our right, a deep canyon filled only with air. It's like the scene before me sucks my eyeballs out of my head trying to grasp with my vision all that is before me. The same thing happens at the Grand Canyon. It's like my mind can't handle the vastness that it sees.

By mid day, I gnashed my teeth into a brutal head wind while I cranked up long, nasty climbs. We never got a break. The wind howled. We dipped down into the Gorge only to suffer a miserable climb to get out of it. We lost 800 feet of vertical in 90 seconds only to take 45 minutes to climb back up again. It was enough to discourage anyone, but on a bike tour, no one feels sorry for you or cares about your plight. Denis and I kept pushing into that inland gale. Riding with Denis was good because he and I never complained about our situation. Sure, we loved tailwinds and long down hill descents, but when it came to brutal climbs and head winds or rain--we knew the score. Helen Keller said it best with her statement that there is no security in nature—no guarantees of an easy ride.

At one point, we pedaled downhill against a ferocious blast coming up from the valley. It demoralized us. It wearied our souls. No escape! We endured and kept on keeping on.

At times like that, I was not having fun. I asked myself what in the devil was I doing? The muscle, guts and determination it took to keep going exceeded most peoples' comprehension. But, if you're pedaling a bike, you can't quit, give up or cry. You are forced, or at least, you force yourself to do something--and the only 'something' is to pedal onward--up the hill or across the windswept flats.

Whatever it is within my mind that makes me love to do this bike touring also makes me accept myself in the place I find myself in the world. I deal with whatever is happening and move forward.

Therefore, bicycle adventure and life struggles enjoy a lot in common.

We crossed over the Flaming Gorge Dam. A large blue lake backed up for dozens of miles. We climbed from 5,000 feet back up to 8,000 feet. After climbing for an hour, we stopped at a campsite overlooking the lake that gave us a glowing sunset, aromatic juniper trees and chirping birds. An older couple sat reading their books in the campsite 30 meters from us. They gave us a loaf of bread for dipping in our soup and rice-bean dinners.

To say the least, hunger raged within us. Sitting there, we faced the lake while we devoured food. In many ways, our dining table offered us a view that rich people enjoy. Don't you ever wonder what it's like to be rich and have a mansion on a lake where you can watch fabulous sunsets over the water? That's one of the joys of bicycle adventure--I've had my tent flaps turned toward some of the most amazing sights in the world: Mount Everest, Wall of China, Yosemite, Great Ocean Road in Australia, Inca Trail, Denali, Cotapoxi in South America, Antarctica, Parthenon, Oracle of Delphi and a hundred more. Perhaps, that makes me a wealthy man.

Nothing to brag about because it was all fleeting--but still, my eyes enjoyed the visions--and I didn't have to be rich to relish them.

After dinner, the sky darkened. Exhaustion struck us! We felt beat to death.

"Bon nuit Denis," I said.

"Bon nuit Frosty," Denis said.

I don't even remember my head hitting the pillow. Sleep engulfed me like a pleasant feeling of joy in all my cells. Most likely, they were happy to be at rest after I had 'forced' them to fight through a day of mean, nasty, cruel, harsh, dastardly, rotten, merciless, awful, terrible, mind bending, teeth gnashing, howling--HEAD WINDS!

Thank you Helen Keller for sharing your power. Yes! Bicycling is a daring adventure!

CHAPTER 12 — BECAME PART OF DARKNESS

"I went to the woods because I wished to live deliberately, to confront only the essential facts of life, and see if I could not learn what it had to teach, and not, when I came to die, discover that I had not lived. I did not wish to live what was not life, living is so dear; nor did I wish to practice resignation, unless it was quite necessary. I wanted to live deep and suck out all the marrow of life."

Henry David Thoreau

"You'll find Vernal about 15 minutes down the road," a local man said, itching his gray bearded chin.

Many people operate under the influence of an automobile. Fifteen minutes means 15 miles. For us, on a bike, with fully loaded panniers, it might mean an hour or maybe two and a half hours depending on a hill climb. If it is a nasty nine to twelve percent grade, it could be four hours of exhausting, sweat-soaking, food munching and leg busting work. On a bicycle tour, time slows down to a manageable pace. What most folks cover in an hour, takes us all day.

Every hill has a price and every down hill coast possesses its joy. But it all costs a physical payment. Yesterday, I struggled with those head winds and unending hills. I cursed at the universe when I saw the road drop 1,000 feet to the Flaming Gorge Dam--because I could see the climb back up again. In fact, from 5,400 feet to 8,400 feet. That's a 3,000 foot climb, inch by inch, pedal stroke by pedal stroke...slow, arduous climbing.

Why do we do it? I remembered that man in Glacier National Park feeling sorry for us. Another lady said she wouldn't want to go through what we went through, but she wouldn't mind being in shape like we were. I wondered if this country with its ease and convenience, with its microwaves, cars and escalators, fast foods and one-hour photos is losing its will or the glory that comes from a singular quest. Millions must love the quest.

Look at them glued to the TV set for the NFL, NBA, NHL, baseball, soccer and tennis. That doesn't include HBO and Internet junkies who sit in front of the monitor for hours playing games or looking for something to challenge them.

Is struggle no longer an American rite of passage? Beats me! I like the struggle for the moments of serenity it brings me, for the spiritual joy and connection to the earth, for the rhythms of life that course through my body, and, for the simple pleasures of riding a bicycle. For me, to miss a campfire and the starlit sky above me with the big dipper sparkling against the ink black of space--well--that is not something to be missed. There in the sky, through the pine trees, a shooting star! Forever, a special moment in my mind.

John Muir said, "When you pick up a rock, you realize it's hitched to everything else in the universe."

When we pulled out of the campground, the host lady said, "You're pretty ambitious this early in the morning."

"What doesn't kill me on this mountain," I said, "will make me stronger."

"Better you than me," she said.

As I stood on the pedals, I couldn't help but agree-yes-me better than her! What a privilege to be able to take on such a quest across the whole country on the toughest, most mountainous of routes.

The climb proved rough, ever upward through the pines and into the aspen groves, just waiting to turn into fall colors. Those shimmering golds and sunshine yellows would soon paint the woods in autumn magic.

We saw a family of mule deer hopping across the highway. What a grand sight seeing them bound away! That's the special significance about riding along in the silence. Years ago, I rode in New Mexico on Route 72 near Parker at dusk. It had been a blistering hot day and my body felt like a dishrag that had cleaned out a pot of greasy spaghetti and was hung over the top tube to dry.

My chances of finding a stream for a bath were like a hummingbird flying to the moon.

Nonetheless, it had been a good day. Red flowering cacti filled the air with their elegant perfume scent and pink cloud-lace sliced the heavens into confetti streamers while the sun lit up billowing thunderheads that boiled toward the last light. Their tails faded into the eastern darkness. Saucer-like clouds skidded across the sky to the south of me.

Nearing a small town named Bouse, I stopped at a closed gas station and parked my bike against the side of the cracked, plaster wall of the building.

"Might as well check the spigot to see if I can get a bath," I said, kneeling by the pumps. "I'll be darned! Water!"

I grabbed my soap, razor and towel. The water shot out of the faucet full blast. I soaked myself, clothes and all. After soaping up my shirt, shorts and socks, I shaved my face. As usual, my neck resembled a bloody dog fight after the razor had done its business. No matter what the ads say about shavers, they can rip a man's throat to ribbons.

Nevertheless, my body tingled at the new-found clean feeling on my skin. After rinsing away the soap from my shorts and shirt, I stepped into clean clothes. I hung my wet tights, socks and jersey onto the back of my pack for quick drying, and loaded my water bottles.

Bouse featured ramshackle buildings on flat desert sands. I cranked into the cool evening air. A mile out of town, I scanned the road for a campsite. My tires made the only sound as stillness crept over the land. A few birds flew over the sagebrush and the thunderheads had darkened with the fading light.

I don't like being on the road at twilight. Too dangerous!

"Come on, where's a place to camp?" I complained out loud. "I'm out in the middle of nowhere, and I can't find a place to sleep."

In the distance, not more than a hundred yards away, I saw a building.

"Bingo!" I said. "That looks like home tonight."

In minutes, I would have my tent set up behind the building and be cooking dinner. That highway was deserted, which meant a quiet night's sleep.

Just then, a coyote loped along the highway off to my right 30 yards away. He looked intent on something that caught his eye. I pressed harder on the pedals. He continued along, not hearing or noticing me. He ran ghostlike in the twilight shadows. His gray body with tan and black hair melted him into the fading light like your black bedspread vanishes when you turn off the light in your room. He was as quiet as the air.

As I followed him, he veered toward the high side of the shoulder near a bush. When he approached it, a jackrabbit shot out of the cover, headed straight down the side of the pavement. The coyote changed from loping gear to Warp Factor two. Every muscle in his body coiled. The stillness was broken by a cloud of dust from his feet and the race was on. The rabbit did a three step hoppity, hoppity, hoppity hop, then ran four strides like a dog, then three more short half steps, and back to running like a dog. At the same time, the coyote, with his nose cutting into the air like an F-16 jet and his tail streaming behind him, edged closer and closer. About the second the coyote was about to open his mouth and grab the rabbit, the speedster turned on a dime and shot left across the highway in front of me. Mr. Coyote pulled his teeth back into his mouth and executed a 90 degree turn. From a dead stop of zero, the coyote accelerated again to high speed. Again, the rabbit raced ten yards along the highway and made another right turn. Mr. Coyote closed quickly like Tom Cruise in "Top Gun" did on his MIG quarry.

On the right side of the road again, the rabbit, followed less than a few steps behind by the coyote, leaped across a shallow culvert. Big mistake! As he sailed over the ditch, the dark figure of the coyote leaped faster and higher through the air--like a heat-seeking missile homing in on its prey. In midair, the coyote's teeth reached down and clamped onto the rabbit. When they fell to earth, the rabbit screamed a death cry. It was like a woman going through childbirth—helpless, and suffering from the pain. Then silence!

Upon pedaling up to the spot, I saw the coyote, with rabbit in his mouth, become part of the darkness.

So yes, on my bicycle, I'll agree with the lady, "Better you than me!"

At the top of the 8,400 foot pass, we dripped like a horses at the Kentucky Derby. But soon, the road began its descent. Not only did we have a cool breeze, but gravity became our motors. It took over and like kids on a free ride at the fair, a smile blazed across our faces. That road carried us 10 miles downhill. It felt like forever. In front of us a desert of pancake-layered mountains of red, tan and gray rock. Barren rock dominated the landscape.

We passed through Pre-Cambrian, Cretaceous, Jurassic, Colombian, and more epochs of time. The land changed. I took a hit of water and an apple. On the sides of a mountain, a group of archeologists dug for fossils.

"Call me when you find the fossil that connects humans with the monkeys," I yelled. "I'm looking for one of my long lost uncles."

They laughed.

Down the road plunged into a great red and gray canyon with rock formations that defied description. One looked like a battleship. Another sandstone formation looked like a pile of buffalo dung. A third looked like a six stack of pancakes with the same tan color. In many cases juniper pines grew right out of the solid rock. Maroon and camel tans collided with the pale blue sky. We kept pedaling in profound wonder--mesmerized by the desolate beauty.

In Vernal, we stocked up on food. Denis gave me a lecture over buying a bag of fried potatoes from the grocery store. He spoke about the trans-fat content and the harm it caused. Usually, I'm strict with my nutrition

99 percent of the time. But once in awhile I eat junk food. Heck, why not? I'm on an adventure. One can't be too pure. Besides, perfection is a fault in itself.

In that small town, we moved through a crowded city with autos and people. Fast food joints and shopping malls dominated the scene. Everywhere—Wendys, Pizza Hut, McDonalds, Arbys, Burger King, Dominoes Pizza, Taco Bell, 7-11, Circle K, K-Mart, Target, Sears, Blimpie's, BlackJack Pizza, Long John Silver, Red Lobster and a dozen more! One thing about modern times, such sameness has destroyed the regional flavor of every corner of our country. Cities maintain redundancies because the buildings that house those retail outlets duplicate ad nauseam. Such a pity! What made it more distressing stemmed from our being out in the middle of nowhere for the last week, so much so, the city annoyed us. However, we needed to replenish our food supplies.

From Vernal, we headed east on Route 40 toward Dinosaur 35 miles away. We pedaled through hot, flat terrain. We welcomed the change after two days of hills and head winds.

Dinosaur National Monument superseded our expectations! Anyone who has seen Jurassic Park will love the exhibits on dinosaurs that lived on this continent more than 165 million years ago. Big T-Rex and Stegosaurus and the first reptiles that took to the air--it's all there. One of the more interesting aspects we gained from the monument was the knowledge that this planet has had five great extinction sessions as they are called. When life first blossomed from the primordial muck, it took many forms as it evolved on land and in the air. From records that are becoming more clearly documented in this scientific age, the fourth extinction session occurred when an asteroid hit the earth causing a nuclear winter. A cloud blanketed the earth and stopped sunlight from getting through--enough to kill the food chain and that's what ended the dinosaurs' reign. From their time, 97 percent of life on this planet suffered extinction. Only three percent of what was left--evolved into the next great living groups that flourished until the last ice age when 95 percent of those creatures died off. From that remaining five percent, our latest 30 million species has sprung, including humanity. To grasp that time span is amazing. In geologic time, we humans have been on the earth for about three seconds. My bet is that we'll be gone in another three seconds of geologic time. The universe won't burp by the time we're extinct.

The more sobering aspect learned while at the exhibit is the fact that the sixth extinction session tumbles forward right now. Guess who is driving it? You're right if you guessed the culprit: erectus, hairless, naked, laughing, crying, crazy primates, i.e., humans. We've become too clever for our own good. Human beings overpopulate the planet by an amazing rate of 77 million net gain of us each year. We're causing the extinction of thousands and soon, tens of thousands of our fellow creatures and plants.

The 21st century, I suspect, will be horribly consequential for our species. And, unfortunately, the other species can only hang on as we leave them smaller and smaller space to live and reproduce. At this time, we, for example, kill 100 million sharks per year, so many that several species live on the brink of extinction. Not only that, we spread our poisons in the air, on the land and in the water--all over the globe. There's no end to our fecundity either. Only nature will put a stop to us via disease, famine, flood, war and climate changes. I suspect that it is a race between economic forces that will break down nature so it can't operate. Or, nature will decimate us down via environmental consequences. One way or the other, we lose and this planet will make us a mere footnote, much like the dinosaurs.

The area was once an ancient seabed, and then a tropical paradise for the dinosaurs and then the great asteroid collision. From there the ice age killed most life.

Now, there's a history of it all in the rocks.

We pushed into the desert's hot, unrelenting sun. Sandstone rock hills spread out across the landscape in front of us. Only bushes and desert grass grew in clumps.

At one point, the highway department had erected a monument to a bunch of Spanish priests led by Father Dominguez, who in 1750, explored Utah and Wyoming, and tried to convert the 'savage' Indians away from their 'inferior' religions.

It never fails to intrigue me that different religions attempt to convert other people to their 'right' or only one 'true' religion. I smile when I see two boys in black pants, white shirts and ties as they ply neighborhoods in America and South America in order to 'convert' others to their 'only' right religion accepted by the 'only' god of the universe.

I have to wonder if God is a Jew, Catholic, Protestant, Hindu, Buddhist, Muslim, Christian, Hari Krishna, Confucian, Dreamland of the Aboriginals of Australia, or anyone of a thousand other religions I don't even know about. Which one is God? God must be scratching his/her/its head daily as God watches the human drama unfold. Of course, it's God's fault because he/she never speaks to us—it only shows signs--and only guys like the Pope, Billy Graham, Jerry Falwell, Oral Roberts, Moses (Charlton Heston), and Robert Schuller have the ears, or is it their egos, big enough to hear or see God's profound utterances?

In this continuing deistic question, I discovered a reasoned definition of God based on my 50 years of study at all locations around the globe. God, I think, is an "emerging creative energy" that creates order in the universe. It destroys, too! It creates and destroys--all in a random chance manner. Nothing means anything to this energy. It's dumb, deaf, blind and without purpose. It simply is. We think we're its most advanced creation. However, all our cries for mercy mean nothing to it. Not then and not now.

Good, bad or indifferent, this creative energy rules the universe in its meaninglessness. We try to pin it with love, caring and purpose, but it never answers us.

We have special people who seem to have a direct line to that energy, i.e., all the great religious leaders like Jesus, Mohammed, Buddha, Moon, etc., but, in reality, they too are as unknowing of that energy as we are.

This planet is one of its more profound creations and it too one day will vanish in a cosmic black hole or our star will become a supernova.

One way or the other, this planet and all life will exist no longer. This 'energy' doesn't give a twit because it doesn't have a brain, or thoughts, or motive.

However, I am delighted that I got to go along for the ride for one brief shining moment. I was born to good parents, with enough brain power and chance for education, to be able to experience an incredible life of thinking and travel. Who should I thank?

God?

That's fine for what it means to me. I'll thank my lucky stars. However, even with my basic understanding of the god-energy, I'm thankful for living and have a spiritual appreciation for this "emerging creative energy of the universe."

Others may enjoy another take on the concept of God. Good for them! Whatever fits a person's spiritual path brings validity and meaning to each person. I support all 6.6 billion human interpretations of God on the planet.

When we reached Dinosaur, Colorado, we met a bicycling Japanese student, Nariuki, traveling from Portland to Denver. We took some pictures of dinosaurs and headed to a park where they provided a pavilion and water.

The Japanese kid ate like a starving dog. He spoke a bit of English and featured a smile pasted to his face. He felt afraid that he would get shot in America. In fact, all Japanese think that they will get killed in America with all the guns and killings. I told him that it was mostly in the inner cities and ghettoes after dark. He was safe out on the road.

We prepared dinner with soup first. We tried to fix his burner but it was broken with a plugged line. I had the soup boiling and poured it directly from the fire into his pan. He immediately started sucking it down like it was a cold beer on a 95 degree day. I tried to sip mine three minutes later and it still burned my lips. He must have scalded his mouth and throat, but it didn't seem to faze him. Next, Denis offered him noodle casserole. Nariuki whipped out his chop sticks and shoveled the food into his starved, lion-like mouth. Again, it boiled hot off the burner. He smiled. Denis offered him a banana. He sucked that down like a glass of juice.

For breakfast the next morning, Nariuki ate a white hamburger bun and American cheese. Denis offered him oatmeal and I cut him a banana. When Denis poured the hot water into his pan, Nariuki looked like a nervous race horse ready to burst from the gate. Denis put his hand out to calm him down.

"Let the oatmeal soak up the water," Denis said.

"Yeah," I said. "Let me cut these bananas."

Two minutes later, Denis said, "Eat!"

The chopsticks flew like a pair of helicopter whirling blades. I mean, this guy mowed down the pan of oatmeal like locusts charging over a wheat field. He left nothing. His mouth sounded like a grinding combine. I eat pretty fast, but I was like a tortoise to the hare when it came to Nariuki. Denis fixed him two PB & Js, and they vanished in the blink of an eye. He cut a peach in half. Nariuki vacuumed it out of his hand in a twinkling.

This twenty-one year old college student had talked about how dangerous America was, but I felt I might lose a finger or a piece of my hide feeding that human garbage disposal.

We took several pictures and he stood right up to me like I was a long lost friend--when, I could easily be his father's age.

I took off as Denis finished breakfast. Route 64 to Rangely rolled slightly downhill with a few climbs. Morning sunshine filled a cobalt sky. Shadows played across the land and flowers brightened to the coming day. Several deer grazed along the road and when they turned to look at me, their 10 inch high ears blazed with the back-lighting from the sun. Miles later, pronghorn antelope raced across the road. A meadowlark issued her familiar call.

My legs pounded the pedals and all was right with my world. I made Rangley in 90 minutes. Big-nosed derricks sucked black gold out of the ground everywhere. It was hard to imagine that the USA burns 20 million barrels every 24 hours, 365 days a year and the world burns 80 million barrels per day without end. How the heck do they get it out of the ground that fast?

Denis caught up with me and we turned south on Route 139 up a wide river valley. Tan and red rocks in birthday cake layers stood like sentinels as we passed through the valley. Several hours later, we began a 3,000 foot climb to Douglas Pass at 8,200 feet. The grade hit 14 percent in some places--which meant my legs worked hard. But no worries, because at that point, my legs felt strong. I really didn't feel the climbs. They became effortless.

While pedaling, I watched Denis come from behind with his slow even-powered strokes. He soon passed me. I felt content knowing I would never have his or John Brown's leg strength. When you get with guys of their athletic caliber, you feel humbled, but you're like a little kid and thankful they would let you play in their ball game.

The pass kept going up and I thanked my legs for being so strong. At some points, the climb challenged us with 15 percent grades. I couldn't help thinking about John Brown's daily battle with cancer. He struggled with chemotherapy and radiation. What did he think about--living or dying? What about his kids and wife? My climb was nothing compared to his battle. I was so angry at the universe for striking him down with cancer--but it did no good. I could only offer my hopes for his best possible recovery.

At the top, the wind blew and the road took a nose dive through the green of the canyon below us. It cooled at the top. We snapped pictures and headed down.

"We've coasted ten miles," Denis said after he finally put his foot down.

"That's easier than going up," I said.

The valley led us down and out of the mountains until I stopped with a flat tire. I picked up a metal sliver. While fixing my tire, I realized the chain and two chain rings needed replacing in Moab.

In Loma, we hit a deserted park, cooked dinner and passed out. We had traveled 95 miles.

"Ding, ding, ding, ding," a set of railroad bells chimed into the night.

Before I knew it, I thought a train was rushing through my brain. It whistled and then blew through my tent like a tornado. I woke up thinking I was going to be run over. Just as quickly, it passed 30 yards away with a clickity, clickity, clickity....

Two more trains raced through, but I felt safe except for the noise. As luck would have it, we caught a misbegotten road out of Loma on Route 6 that wasn't on the map. It headed west to an intersection with I-70 where we would connect with the Cisco exit 212. The road turned from asphalt to broken patched concrete, to gravel, and finally, to sand. We passed a couple of junkyard homes. One big bus stood out in the field and people lived in it. Nothing but desert stretched to flat top mountains in the distance. Sand and sagebrush covered the landscape with multi-colored mountains on the horizon.

Within miles, the road became a one-track sand trail. It broke up and was grown over by weeds. I-70 rolled along directly on our left and people drove by looking at us. Some waved or honked. We passed the Westwater exit. The road grew worse as we passed exit 220. We had eight miles to go to Cisco by following a treacherous dirt road. After a few miles, we decided to throw the gear and bikes over the fence and ride on I-70 for the last five miles.

We stripped the bikes and passed them over the fence. Denis was not in too good a humor about it, but he was soon happy to be on smooth highway. It was good to leave the sand trail because we were beating up our panniers on the rough road.

Riding like that reminded me of when we rode in Bolivia over a nasty corrugated road for 500 miles over 12,000 and 15,000 foot passes. The road was so bumpy, our butts bled from the constant pounding. Our hands shook from holding the bars that vibrated with the wheels hitting the corrugations in the gravel. It was so bad, we tried to ride the animal trails alongside the railroad tracks that paralleled the road, but our pedals struck the embankment and tumbled us down the incline. We pedaled through pretty scenery with vibrant green tundra grass growing up the mountains which gave way to solid gray rock that led to immense pointed peaks. But it was the most miserable riding I can ever remember. When we reached asphalt near Lake Titicaca, we knelt down and kissed the cement. Without a doubt, South America is one of the greatest bicycle adventures on the planet— but also one of the toughest.

We reached the Cisco exit and stopped to rest under a blazing sun. It was a sinister fireball in the sky--incessant, eternal, giving light, but cooking us and that arid region under its unrelenting heat.

Just as we headed southward along the highway to Cisco, Utah, a man with a load of cantaloupe melons and watermelons pulled off the Interstate. He pulled over to the side of the exit and stopped near a garbage can which had a lid on it.

I pedaled back toward him. All I could think of was a big fat juicy watermelon cascading down my parched throat.

"What's the chance a thirsty cyclist could buy a few melons off you?" I asked.

"Sure," he said. "What would you like?"

"I'd like a watermelon and a cantaloupe."

"I've got a Persian you might like to try," he said as he lifted several fat ones from the trailer.

"What's the damage?" I said.

"Three dollars," he said.

We put them on the trash can lid and cut the watermelon open. Seconds later, we proceeded to slurp our mouths into big smiles with cool, wet, tasty, delicious watermelon. The rush of sugar and cool watermelon tantalized our taste buds. I cut strip after strip, and gobbled it into my mouth. It was like a dream trip eating a cool melon out in the middle of a hot desert. Every mouthful exploded with sweet sensation on my tongue. It made me laughing happy. I think Denis thought I had lost my mind, but he was smiling, too. That was a peak moment. I swear that it was the greatest watermelon I had ever eaten in my life.

We made ourselves fat and sick on watermelon before packing the other two into our panniers.

Off again, we pedaled across the wasteland of sagebrush for several miles until we came into the town of Cisco. It was a railhead for years for the goods in Moab, Utah that connected to the markets in Grand Junction, Colorado. Now, it had two broken down homes, sod houses, outhouses, wrecked cars, strewn junk plus trash scattered everywhere. The post office was a 9'x9' wooden structure with weeds growing everywhere. Once again, I felt saddened to see junk left over by humans who had no respect for the land.

At times like that, I wish I had Bill Gates' $50 billion. I'd go about the country on a crusade for cleaning up trash, wrecked cars, and abandoned homes. I'd pay the people who owned the land to clean up their junk and put it back to the way nature made it. With $50 billion,

I'd be a huge force for good across this land. Instead, Bill built a $20 million dollar mansion. He needs it to house his wife and kids, but I would have used the money for restoring nature. In his defense, he and billionaire Warren Buffet joined forces to contribute to kids and health programs around the world.

For me and my spare $50 dollars, I'll continue my own dream by cleaning up every campsite I come across and picking up trash wherever I find it. At a minimum, I'm doing something.

We snapped a few pictures and headed back into the desert. The road led down toward the cavernous red and tan colored flat-top mountains south of us. It resembled a ribbon in the wind or a snake appearing and vanishing before us. We had no idea where it took us but trusted it led toward Moab.

Down it dropped into the canyon. We rolled along the churning, gray silt waters of the Colorado River. From our high road overlooking the peaks and cliffs, we descended them. It was like riding into the intestines of nature--all twisted, narrow, moving and colorful. Layers and layers of sediment rock rose from the ground like multi-layered wedding cakes. Red, tan, gray, purple, brown, burgundy, some thick--some thin, layers of rock billions of years old surrounded us. We rode at the bottom of an ancient sea. From that seabed, the Colorado River cut a mighty living sculpture--a magical visual extravaganza—more profound with every turn in the road.

We followed the road with 1,000-foot vertical rock walls rising right up from the pavement. The jagged rock walls flew up to the sky where red rock clashed with blue sky. Solid rock collided with blue nothingness. Who won the clash? We did because our eyes marveled at the formations. Along our path, giant clumps of sunflowers bloomed yellow petals and brown inner circles. Rocks tumbled down the mountain sides and lay in all sorts of positions as if a child had played with alphabet blocks and left them scattered about the playroom.

We rode to a point where the valley opened wide. Great spires and tubular columns shot into the sky. Some of the mountains resembled battleships plowing through the deep blue ocean sky. Others looked like smokestacks on huge factory buildings. Other formations, all in rusted red colors looked like pipe organs in a church--only the size of an entire mountain. The music they played could only be heard by our eyes.

After several miles, the canyon narrowed again and we hugged vertical rock walls on our left and rushing waters on our right.

Denis decided to make Moab and I decided to camp under the canyon walls. He kept rolling downward when I turned off into a campsite along the river. "I'll meet you in town in the morning," I said. Above me, the last light of the day played across the 1,000-foot rock walls above me. My sandy campsite featured overgrown bushes off the river. I heard the ripples of the current as it passed by my site.

Sharing the spot with me, Jack, a 25 year old engineer, had hiked over the Continental Divide carrying a 90 pound pack. From there, he jumped into his single-man raft and floated 135 miles down the Colorado on his way to California. His pack would have killed me in five miles. We ate dinner and hit the hay.

That night, the canyon sky changed from blue to silver to pink to black. Once the sun set, the rock cliffs mingled with that magic sky. Without note or fanfare, one by one, stars twinkled in the enchanting night sky.

The only sound I heard with my last moment of consciousness that day came from the rippling of the river current.

CHAPTER 13 — STINKS LIKE HELL

"Tentative efforts lead to tentative outcomes. Therefore give yourself fully to your endeavors. Decide to construct your character through excellent actions and determine to pay the price of a worthy goal. The trail you encounter will introduce you to your strengths. Remain steadfast.... and one day you will build something that endures; something worthy of your potential."

Epictetus
Roman Philosopher

Some kind of strange bird chirped me awake in the morning. I broke the tent open to see a 1,000 foot wall of red sandstone rock blazing with morning sunlight. Jack, my new camping friend, sat back on the sand looking up at the sky. The sound of swirling waters of the river seeped through the bushes. In the rock wall above me, a hole much like a wide end of a megaphone blasted out to the world. From many places, the rock featured black painted zebra-like strips dropping down from cracks where water had seeped and stained it.

Jack and I ate breakfast. He wanted to write me so I gave him my address. He wanted to be a writer. Maybe I should have dissuaded him to save him from years of frustration. Becoming a writer harbors more hardship and rejection than any other job on the planet.

At the Poison Spindle bike shop in Moab, I replaced two chain rings and a chain on my bike.

Denis showed up and we found a campsite in town. It featured wall to wall motor homes and tents packed into a giant gravel parking lot. So much for a wilderness vacation!

From there, we pedaled to Arches. I bought Denis "DESERT SOLITAIRE" by Edward Abbey. It's a book about Arches and the surrounding area from 30 years ago. It's funny, irreverent, spiritual and full of joy.

What was going to be an easy day of sightseeing turned out to be 41 miles round trip with a 5,000 foot climb. It took us two miles to climb to the park's entrance. Riding out of Moab does not prepare a cyclist for the gargantuan splendor waiting at the Arches entrance. After crossing the Colorado River, the road swept upward like a Frisbee on a long arcing flight. Around the first towering stone wall of red sandstone, a gallery of spires and pinnacles, in odd and grotesque shapes, seemed to peer down at us. It was like riding up a New York street with the Empire State Building rising straight up until we couldn't tell how high it was because it was beyond our perspective.

We jumped into a line of 20 cars waiting to get into the park. Even a September weekend made for a visitor-plagued madhouse. Lots of French, German, Swiss, British, Aussie, Japanese, Dutch and Kiwis visited the park. I met another Japanese couple who were afraid to come to America because they feared getting shot. I told them it wasn't that bad if they avoided visiting Detroit, Los Angeles, Chicago, Atlanta and New York inner city areas at night! Beyond that, they would be relatively safe except on a major city freeway at rush hour! Also, they shouldn't go down by the border where drug runners would shoot them on sight.

As I stood there telling them that America was safe and that they weren't in any danger, I remembered an incident I lived through two years ago. Gary and I, with our ladies, had finished dancing at "Swing Time in the Rockies" at the Holiday Inn on I-70 and Chambers Road. We decided to go to an International House of Pancakes on Peoria Street for a late night breakfast. We walked into the place and sat down within 90 seconds. Suddenly, outside, shots rang out in the parking lot. Two guys wielding 357 magnums chased and fired at each other out front. As can be imagined, everyone in the restaurant dove to the floor and covered their heads. Minutes later, the cops came and chased after the villains who had done the shooting.

We ordered and ate our breakfast while the cops stood guard outside. When we walked out an hour later, my rear tire had been blown to pieces. After looking around the car, I discovered a large bullet hole in the side of my car door.

"My car's been shot!" I yelled.

"Where?" Gary asked.

"Right here," I said, pointing. "They shot my poor defenseless car."

"Better your car than you," Gary said.

As I stood there talking to the Japanese, I remembered bicycling in Japan in 1985. Out of a city of more than 25 million in Tokyo and its suburbs, they had four killings in 1985 as of November of the year. Four in a year! No wonder Japanese think it's dangerous in America.

There are seven killings a week in Detroit and one or more in Denver every couple of days. Scratching my head, I had to agree that America is a dangerous place--in the cities, on our nation's highways and in our homes. We kill ourselves at the rate of 23,000 handgun murders per year. We kill 44,000 on the highways. When all the violent movies and TV shows are thrown in, which the Japanese watch, yes, Mrs. Jones, the USA is a dangerous place. If they watch Jerry Springer and Howard Stern, they must think we are totally Looney Toons.

Starting from the front gate of Arches astounded us. The road climbed along a crescent vertical wall of grandiose proportions. Great rock columns that jutted into view from the distance now stood above us. One hundred thousand ton rocks, looking like fresh loaves of bread dough ready for the oven—rested on top in various shapes. Three such rock columns rose 500 feet above us and looked like three penguins waddling across the sky. We pedaled under them like two fleas scurrying under the Statue of Liberty.

The road serpentined through four switch-backs and kept us sweating all the way to a place called Park Avenue. In a one million year swipe of erosion, heat, water and freezing--two walls of rock formed what could easily be mistaken for Park Avenue in New York. Rock skyscrapers complete with 'rock' satellite dishes on the top rose into the sky. On the left, one 50 ton rock balanced on the thin top of the wall. The next wind storm should knock it off.

We hit the road again for a direct view of a rock that resembled a giant church organ five hundred feet tall. To its left were three towering columns of rock that looked like three women talking to each other. They named it "The Three Gossips."

What created those colossal formations and what made them stand out? Simple: Entrada Rock. It was a form of sandstone that stood up after the salt deposits liquefied and eroded. An ancient sea that once covered the region deposited them. The weaker materials washed away--leaving Amazing formations.

Many places featured hobgoblins sitting on the tops of thick 500 foot walls called fins. In several places it looked like a shark's fin prowled the sky. In another, the three stooges, Larry, Curly and Moe, caused mischief across the landscape.

In many of the spires, it looked like someone had poured water and sand together, like at the beach to create a lumpy castle. But in this case, the spires stood hundreds of feet high.

In one place, nature had carved out a long finger as if she was flipping someone the bird. Another shape looked like Jonah the Whale while another was the spitting image of Dumbo the Elephant.

Further into the park about 14 miles, we passed a valley of petrified sand dunes. At the end of the dunes, we pedaled up on a most unlikely shape. A rock in the profile of a large soup spoon stood out from the rest. It perched on a narrow handle of rock. At more than 80 tons, it could crash any moment. It was called "Balanced Rock." If the slightest wind blew; the spoon face would fall. Its little brother, "Chip off the old Block," fell in 1990. From there, an entire group of formations, called the "Garden of Eden," stretched for a mile. In that span, a dozen arches opened their holes to the blue sky. It was the "Windows" section of the park--and highly dramatic.

We backtracked and made our way to "Delicate Arch." A two mile hike brought us to an amphitheater where a single arch stood five stories high on the edge of a cliff. It was as if someone had decided to place it there for no other reason than to trick the human eye. A crowd of 50 snapped pictures when I walked down to the center of the arch and looked back up at them. I don't know what made me do it, but I clasped my hands to my mouth and megaphoned, "Friends, Romans and countrymen, lend me your ears....I come to bury Caesar not to praise him....for whether it is nobler in...."

That brought a small applause from the crowd. Usually, I'm a quiet, taciturn, and unassuming man. It must have been the moment that spurred me to ancient Shakespearean oratory.

"More, more," the hungry crowd yelled.

"No, No, NO!" I yelled back. "I am but a humble man, quiet....reaching out to the world for truth."

"Boo," they screamed back. "We want more!"

Demurely, I called back, "I've lost my voice."

"Hang that guy to the nearest arch!" one man screamed.

"Touchy, touchy," I said, sensing the venomous crowd rising against me.

Fame is but a fleeting feather on a delicate wind. You're a hero one moment and a goat the next. I decided to get out of the limelight before the first tomato made its way down to me.

Further toward the end of the park, we passed what appeared to be an NFL football stadium full of the faces and bodies of fans. Their colors consisted of salmon and white. For so many, they were awfully quiet. It was yet another display of rocks created by nature to give the appearance of people in a stadium. Amazing!

Landscape Arch lay at the end of the road. We hiked in a mile through a narrow canyon of finned rock as if we walked through a school of sharks. After twenty minutes, perhaps the most exquisite arch in the park stretched before us.

Landscape Arch may not be dramatic or powerful, but it supersedes all the others in sheer regal magnitude. A 306 foot arching span of hundreds of tons of rock-- created a rock rainbow across the sky. That's a football field of rock that holds itself up by the pressure of its arc. It could collapse at any time. Yet, it has stood for centuries.

I stood while enjoying the silence. I rested deep in a canyon of rock walls--quiet, with ebbing sunlight, and a white crescent moon slipping into the arch like thread through the eye of a needle. A sense of profound wonder crept through my eyes and settled in my mind. Most of the time in our daily lives, we are assaulted with the wretchedness if not the tyranny of noise. From the morning alarm clock to the beeping of the microwave, we Americans endure horns in traffic to the madness of office din. At home again, the kids scream, dogs bark and the phone rings. I leaned back against the rocks and stared at that rock rainbow. It made no sound, yet it made me hear and see nature's profound creative, patient energy. There is a timeless pulse throbbing through the universe. If we're lucky; we may see its positive handiwork.

Edward Abbey wrote, "If the arches have any significance, it lies, I venture, in the power of the odd and unexpected to startle the senses and surprise the mind out of their ruts and habit, to compel us into a reawakened awareness of the wonderful--that which is full of wonder."

Landscape Arch represents one such place.

We pedaled back to the campground after the park closed. I was in need of a shower. I had so many layers of dried sweat, salt and road grime that I stunk like road-kill. When I took off my helmet, I looked like road-kill. When I took off my shoes, a deadly sort of mustard gas had developed between my toes. My socks could have stopped a herd of buffalo dead in their tracks. I almost passed out. My pits ached with odor. They stunk so bad, I felt guilty walking into the restroom. My crotch, goodness gracious, well, the story of that olfactory assault on civilization cannot be recorded in this decade as I would be arrested and thrown into prison for three consecutive life sentences as a menace to society. My crime: "HE STINKS LIKE HOLY HELL!" Even the mosquitoes wouldn't get near me. My face resembled a greasy wire brush.

My fingernails could supply a shoe polish manufacturer with black dye. My hair, or what was left of it, looked like a family of rats had taken up their nest on my head. Not a pretty sight!

The shower I picked stood in the corner of the building away from the rest of the men. No one came near me. I felt a bit rejected by everyone because my Right Guard had failed after the first day.

That's the one thing about being on a bicycle adventure in the summer and not getting a shower everyday. A person quickly returns to his normal animal heritage. If it weren't for toothpaste, brushes, soap, and TP, we'd all stink like a pack of skunks. We, in fact, are animals--and I'm most aware of that reality on a bike tour.

In many ways, I am a savage--with a ravaging hunger, daily struggle, no sense of time other than sunrise and sunset. I'm out in the rain, heat, dry and cold with no protection. I must accept and endure those faces of nature. Many would say, "Why do you want to suffer like that?"

To me, it's discomfort, yes, but nothing to suffer. How many have bicycled the rain forests of the Amazon? Seen butterflies more exquisite than the nature channels could ever show on film? Felt the sting of a million raindrops? Or heard the call of a Toucan bird? Better yet, felt and heard the awesome roar of the Falls de Gausu in Uruguay? Or, have their hand rubbed by a penguin at the bottom of the world?

Adventure is not always comfortable, but it is still adventure and it is magnificent for those who follow that quest.

"I want to live in this shower!" I yelled out.

"Sounds like a personal problem," some guy responded.

Later, I was as clean as a shiny new dime fresh from the mint. A shower means a whole lot more to touring cyclists than just a shower.

As Thoreau said, "I want to suck the marrow out of the bone...to confront my existence and live deliberately."

While on tour, I confront existence every day on an animal level. It renders a sort of raw power which equals energy.

CHAPTER 14 — EATING A BUG SUCKS

"All men have the stars," he answered, "but they are not the same things for different people. For some, who are travelers, the stars are guides. For others, they are no more than lights in the sky. For poets, they offer inspiration. For others, who are scholars, they are problems. For the businessman, they are wealth. You, and you alone, have stars as no one else has them...I wonder whether the stars are set alight in heaven so that one day each one of us finds his own star again...and now here is my secret, a very simple secret: It is only with the heart that one can see rightly; what is essential to the eye."

The Little Prince
Antoine de Saint Exupery

We 'gassed' up at the City Market with bananas, apples, and energy bars. I felt sad leaving Moab. We stayed three days and witnessed nature's artwork in Arches. We rode the fabled 'Slick Rock Trail' and met dozens of people from around the globe.

I understood why Abbey felt inspired to write his book out there. The sky at sunset last night danced across the heavens much like when you see those Japanese women with six foot streamers at the end of sticks as they swirl them around their heads. The sun blistered the horizon with red flames as it sank below the petrified sand dunes on the western end of Arches. The high rock formations caught the light in a red glow and reflected it as if they were on fire. Booming thunderhead clouds caught the sun's firelight and their billowy white bodies burned crimson against a silver-blue sky. Our shadows grew long across the barren red landscape.

A place like Arches fires the senses, especially the spirit. Perhaps, in our Warp Factor Nine society, we have lost a great deal of our spiritual connection. It may be why so many go about their lives in various degrees of emotional instability. I'm reminded of the school shootings at Columbine in Denver, Colorado, endless wife abuse, child abuse, 16 teen suicides daily in our country, and 22,000 hand gun killings that happen across the USA annually. The undercurrent of pain runs deep in this society at every level.

But for me, Arches gave a sense of the eternal. I knew the sunsets would continue and Landscape Arch would be there each day. The same thing happened to me in the Galapagos Islands. The Blue Footed Booby birds had nested in their nests for hundreds of thousands of years.

Successive generations lived and died before I walked through their plots. Like them, I would pass through, and be gone. The one thing I sensed in the Galapagos was that there is no such thing as "time." It's our invention and when humanity is not around, time vanishes. Only sunrise and sunset. Summer and autumn. Winter and spring. Birth and death. From the black void of nonexistence through a span of living existence to a return to nonexistence. All unstoppable.

That's the nature of life and adventure. It moves along. I can love any part of it, like the watermelon day that was so enthralling, but I can't hold onto the moment. It will pass no matter what I do. Is there any one part of the adventure more important? Sure, the highlights inspire me, but it's the daily pedaling that sustains me. Therefore, I will be delighted with the 'great' moments of the adventure and appreciate all 'little' moments of it.

Rod McKuen, the poet said, "I've been gone a long time now, and along the way, I've learned some things... you have to make the good times yourself; save the little times and make them big times and save the times that are all right for the ones that aren't so good."

Monticello awaited us 57 miles away. It was our goal for the day. The terrain out of Moab featured rounded, tan mountains as if they had been thrown down onto the land like play dough. We rode at 5,000 feet, and even though the road looked flat, as we looked behind us, it kept climbing.

We passed a "hole in the wall home" where a man had dug out a house from one of the great red sandstone mountains. Why and for what he dug it out remains a mystery.

Later, Wilson's Arch appeared alongside the highway. It was a huge, powerful arch. Lots of blue sky could be seen through its "window." We climbed it for several pictures.

Later as we pedaled down the road, a man in a motor home honked his horn in anger while passing us. He was really out of line as there was no reason for his rage. We were in the four-foot bicycle lane, which gave him plenty of room, but he was angry about something. Perhaps he didn't like the way his wife had fixed his eggs that morning--obviously not sunny-side up! What was going on in his mind to blast us with his horn? Were we impeding his travel? Did he think he was the only one allowed to travel the highway? As he passed, Denis raised his finger in a full bird and waved it at the guy who embodied "road rage." Throwing the finger didn't do much, but it made us feel avenged. I personally wouldn't do it in Detroit, however. They'd return a "finger" with bullets.

It's amazing how close we are to our ancestral violence in this society. But if you look at Serbia, India, Pakistan, Afghanistan, Iraq, Sudan, and dozens of other countries, they're all fighting and killing each other across borders. Will we ever transcend our animal nature? I doubt it.

Just one time, I'd like to catch some old geezer like the honking motor home guy in the next parking lot after he had blasted me. I'd verbally climb down his throat and scare the hell out of him. If he was bigger than me, I'd keep my tongue and cower away. Darwin rules! The fact is, if I were bigger, I'd like to beat the hell out of him, but my more socialized character would not do that. But many in this society would and, in fact, do commit violence, because their behavior has no such constraints. I'm probably no better given certain circumstances.

This honking Winnebago incident reminds me of a time when Gary and I pedaled from Boulder to the Maroon Bells in Aspen, Colorado--a week long trip through incredible autumn gold foliage. A guy in a truck nearly ran us over on a curve. We immediately flipped him the bird and yelled at him with more than a few obscenities. We would have gotten into a fight if he had stopped. If I had been attacked, Gary would have jumped in too, to help me. It's that "protect your own" pack mentality. Them versus us! With Gary and me, a total bond of protective brotherhood had developed. We'd die for each other. The same was true for Denis and me. Anybody hurt him; I'd be at their throat in a New York second. We are so sustained by our animal instincts when it comes to the basics of life, which nature created via tribal species group survival dynamics. We, in this society, may think we're civilized, but just turn off the electricity in New York City for a few nights and see what happens. Good grief! We're on the edge!

We pushed a 20 mph head wind for five hours. Around 6:30, we faced 14 miles to Monticello, but again, a large mountain pass reared its ugly head and we had to climb it. We lowered our heads and began a 45 minute climb of 1,000 feet. At the top, we had four more miles to Monticello. The heavens slid into darkness.

The sky! In our rearview mirrors, silver blue brilliance with slivers of white clouds reflected the sun which set and gave a bright strawberry glow to the horizon. It created such a powerful contrast as we pedaled into a tunnel of darkness. Quickly, the night swallowed us. I turned on my red blinking light. As we pedaled, it was still warm, but with the passing minutes the air changed from warm to neutral to cold. It was in those few moments where I felt like I was riding in a dream...effortless, misty, surreal.

We reached Monticello where we found a restaurant. When we walked out from eating a half hour later, night air chilled us. How come so cold? A local man said, "You're at 7,000 feet." We had climbed all day without knowing how far up we had ascended.

We slept on a baseball diamond for the night. In the morning, we found out that Monticello (Italian for "little mountain") was named after Thomas Jefferson's home in Virginia. At breakfast, we met a Scotsman who had biked down from Moab—and, who was proud of his ability to tour with 11 pounds of gear. He owned the barest bicycle I had ever seen. I carried 60 pounds of gear and was prepared for most situations, but yes, it cost me in weight carried. He wore no helmet, glasses, gloves, socks, and enjoyed no mirrors, stove, or plates. He ate everything cold and prided himself in his ability to not drink water. Although I didn't say it, I thought he was a lunatic.

Before pulling out of town, I rode my bike in front of a huge city park flower display. The patch stretched 30 feet long and 20 feet deep with red, yellow, white, black, purple, orange, pink, and many more shades and shapes. Denis took a shot of me lying on my back in front of the display. Throughout the trip, we took dozens of shots in front of flower patches. With the colorful results, I'm going to submit a touring story totally based on flowers from Canada to Mexico.

Pulling out of town, the road rolled straight, smooth and clean. Pretty flat too! We headed for Cortez 64 miles away. Right off the bat, Denis blew a tire. His side wall wore out. Back on the road, I too, suffered a flat. My side wall had worn enough to cut the tire. A quick patch job took care of things.

We had made nine miles in two hours. It was a slow day.

Back on the highway, we rode through a skunk road-kill and, minutes later, a second one. Nothing can stop the horrendous smell of a skunk. One whiff in the old lungs knocks out any sense of joy from the flower patches. I rode along with my mouth open when a winged insect about a half inch long flew in from the side and popped into my mouth. Before I knew it, the bug had slipped past my tongue and slid down my throat. I gagged and tried to hack it up. I choked as my throat closed down. But the bug had gotten too far. Slowly, but surely, it slipped down my throat and out of my control. Down, down, down, it descended into the pit of my stomach.

Just a really sickening feeling eating a bug with its wings, legs and ugly little mouth...not to mention its butt and everything in it! And, me, a vegetarian for heaven sakes! It was probably kicking and screaming all the way down---and, suffocating itself to death as I tried to cough it up.

But, in the end, it went down, and I ended up breaking 27 years of being a vegetarian by eating a bug. As I pedaled along, the idea didn't set well with me, but to get the whole thing out of my mind; I pulled the water bottle out of the cage and guzzled half the contents. From there, I pulled an apple out of my pack to counter the taste of the bug with the taste of an apple. No matter, it was still a yucky feeling eating a bug.

I rode up to Denis, "I ate a bug."

He grinned, "Good protein for you to pedal harder."

"Easy for you to say," I said. "Watch out for those grasshoppers."

Denis smiled.

The rest of the day proved uneventful other than going through Dove Creek which was the "Pinto Bean Capital of the World." The town was a compilation of broken trailer homes and trash. Yes, trash decorated the front lawns of homes from one end of town to the other. It's amazing how some people can choose to live in such squalor in the USA. Even if poor, they could pick up the trash and junk around their dwelling. Instead, they add to it. They must have little to no brains or are so illiterate, they are blind to it. West Virginia and Mississippi are the same way. Race doesn't matter. Whites in West Virginia toss garbage and cars, as well as anything and everything--EVERYWHERE...in the woods, lakes, streams, back yards, cities, and yards. In Mississippi, minorities toss junk from one end of the state to the other. You'd be astounded at the millions of personal garbage dumps on the land across this country. People pour their used oil into the ground by the millions of gallons each year. On a bicycle, I experience a close up look each day and I've ridden across America six times!

Why do they do it? If I put myself into their shoes and walk a mile, I might understand. A friend of mine, Jim told me that when he was growing up, "poverty was like walking through a dark tunnel with no light in sight."

"What do you mean?" I asked.

"You wouldn't understand unless you had been as poor as I was during my childhood," he said. "We only knew poverty and it was normal for us. Not until years later did I see how difficult our lives really were."

If I take that point of view a step further, I would understand why people who throw their garbage outside grew up in that style of life...so, yes, it's normal for them. It is a learned behavior, and if they were born to poverty and trash, they would carry on as if that was normal. And for them, it is normal. For those of us who didn't grow up that way, we may count our blessings because it was the luck of the draw as to who our parents were and how we were raised. Once again, it's that "random chance" deal I spoke of earlier. The same goes for those who were born rich, or good looking, or athletic. It's all the luck of the draw.

We rolled into Cortez. The mountain range near it from the right angle looked like a sleeping Indian princess with a very nice figure. On our way through town, we passed a Golden Corral. It featured a 60 item salad bar of all you can eat.

"Let's set up tents and come back here to eat," I said.

"If you want," Denis replied.

"It's the greatest salad bar in the states," I said. "John Brown and I hit one on our trip across the states in 1986 and made ourselves horribly sick. John ate 11 plates loaded with food. I ate seven plates and nearly killed myself from being stuffed."

"You must practice moderation Frosty," Denis said.

"Yeah, moderation and I go together like mustard on a birthday cake," I said, rolling my eyes.

"This is true," Denis said.

There are two rules to an all-you-can-eat salad bar:

Number 1: Eat something from every offering.
Number 2: Don't make yourself sick by eating too much.

When I entered the corral, my eyes glazed over. More than 60 items begged my attention. Steaming soups, to baked potatoes, to pizza. Salads sparkled under the glass along with hot veggies, rice and fruit displays. The Golden Corral featured a fruit bar, salad bar, pastry bar, entree bar, dessert bar, drink bar and vegetable bar. We had struck the mother lode of eateries.

It's one thing to be hungry, but it's another to be on a bicycle for eight hours and famished. It's worse to be famished because your body doesn't know when to quit. You have to rely on your common sense and brain. But your brain is thinking food and famine, storage and stuffing--so it too is useless for that word called "moderation."

We started at the fruit bar island. We ate fruits of all kinds from around the globe. Pineapple from Australia. Kiwis from New Zealand. Melons from Mexico. Ugly Fruit from Bali. Strawberries from South America. Nectarines from Chile. Watermelons from Mississippi.

The veggie bar offered steaming rice, broccoli, cauliflower, cabbage, corn, green beans, and peas. From there, we attacked the pizza bar and baked potatoes. The empty plates grew on our table...one, two, three, four high....six, seven, eight, nine high.

The waitress stood flabbergasted at our ability to devour every scrap of food in sight.

"We may have to cordon you guys off to protect the rest of our customers," she said. "We don't want to be sued for having two wild men attacking our patrons."

"Just keep the grub coming," I said, looking up from my trough, I mean plate.

Along the way, we gobbled blueberry muffins and chocolate brownies. Our bellies grew and our hunger continued. Next, we hit the cherry cobbler pie and bread pudding--along with creamy smooth chocolate pudding. I had ten helpings and still couldn't stop. Denis brought back cookies and muffins and kept stuffing them into his pack. We were like two little kids trying not to get caught as we stole the cookies. That's it! We were outlaws and should have been shot at dawn or hung at dusk for our skullduggery. However, did we commit a crime? Well, partner, it depends on whether we got caught.

We kept eating desserts, and on to the ice cream soft serve. At that point, my belly looked like it was five months pregnant. I felt uneasy, but no pain. So, I kept going up for more desserts. Couldn't stop myself. Each charge up to the bread pudding was now accompanied by a growing pain, unease and stress as my belly worsened under the deluge of food being dropped down into it.

"You will die," Denis said when I brought back another pudding bowl.

"Happy," I added.

It's an amazing conflict when the mind loses to perceived hunger. I was too full to breathe but couldn't stop going up for more food.

"I must stop with this one," I said, groaning.

Slowly, I scooped up the last of the cherry cobbler out of the pan. I held my swollen belly and sat back. I was done. I had reached my limit. I had eaten so much I was sick.

Denis kept eating. He had a bottomless pit and he was filling it. He kept bringing back cookies and storing them in his pack.

"Good grief Denis," I said. "If we get caught, they will put us in prison for ten years."

Denis got this wild, brazen look in his eyes, "Frosty, would a jury convict two starving bicyclists of stealing a few cookies?"

"A few dozen," I said.

"There's crime everywhere," he said in self-defense. "We are only small time criminals."

The more Denis ate, the faster he ran out of room. He looked like a squirrel. He loaded his cheeks.

As I sat there looking like Java the Hut in Star Wars, I groaned in pain. I wished I could stop, but like a junkie who needed one more fix, I got up and waddled to the dessert bar. The bread pudding could not be denied, or the banana cream pie. Slowly, I loaded the booty into a dish.

Back to the table I waddled.

"Call 911 before I eat this," I told Denis.

They carried me out on a stretcher, at least that's what I thought when I awoke in the morning...lying on my back and looking up at all the bugs running across the top of my tent.

But as Denis said, I staggered out of my chair, more dead than alive, looking like a boa constrictor that had swallowed a pig. Somehow, I had mounted my bike and pedaled a mile to the campsite where I flung my body into the tent and landed on my back where I found myself in the morning.

As the light increased in my tent, I noticed a granddaddy long legs spider crawling across the screen. A dozen skeeters flew along the seam line on the netting. Two small beetles fought each other on the side near the tent pole. A grasshopper sat preening himself. One big ant made his way down the sides of the tent. A red-winged black bird sang a melody.

One thing about camping, you're right down in the grass-- next to and with the bugs. Thankfully, modern day enclosed tents provide total protection from the onslaught of the insect world. But each morning I wake up, they let me know they are around. Especially the mosquitoes. They will eat a man alive in the wilds.

That reminded me about the time I was riding in Alaska when I stopped at a Mountain Man Rendezvous in Glenn Allen. For a week, men and women arrived from all over America to live authentically, like our ancestors. They lived in teepees and wore buckskins. They shot flintlock rifles, threw knives, and exchanged goods with each other. They had arm wrestling contests and moose turd pitching contests. Some guys ate raw fish out of the river. I jumped in with them for a week and had a ball.

But one night, a man named Jack, who stood 6'4" tall and 250 pounds, got drunk. He staggered around the campsite after winning the arm wrestling contest. He had taken his shirt off to scare his opponents, but he didn't scare the mosquitoes. Around midnight, he passed out in his teepee. As can be imagined, there were no screens on the teepee. During the night, squadrons of mosquitoes from all over Alaska landed on his exposed back and made unlimited refueling runs on his blood. In the morning, he had puffed up like a balloon and was in shock from so much blood loss. They air lifted him to Anchorage for an immediate transfusion. He almost died. I must admit, I laughed about it. Damned fool!

As I reclined there in the tent looking at the mosquitoes and thinking about Jack, I felt my stomach. It was surprisingly flat. The pain was gone. I had returned to normal. I felt no hunger whatsoever. It would be awhile before I entered a Golden Corral again.

We packed and headed toward Durango. From flat terrain, we headed back into the mountains. The road responded by climbing up and down, up and down. After a month on the road, our legs had developed a good deal of power. If it was a half hour climb, we clicked into low gear and powered up the mountain side. At the top, we eased over the crest and headed down again. Each hill became another moment toward our goal which was to reach a certain city or national park.

About 20 miles out of Cortez, we climbed to a higher plateau. Ahead of us, an enormous dark gray cloud spit lightning bolts down to the ground every few seconds. A rain squall looking like a liquid silver curtain swept across the mesa in front of us. The contrast of wet green forest and silver liquid sky, touched by intervals of hot white lightning, produced a sensual scene.

As we pedaled toward it, Denis looked at me, "You wanna' go into that?"

"Not me," I said. "Let's stop at the next protected place."

Within a half mile, we saw a tourist stop where a dozen 30 foot long arrows had rained down on a small western town front. The vendor sold Indian jewelry and the arrows definitely attracted attention. Just as we pulled up, it felt like someone had pulled the plug on the rain cloud above us. A rat-a-tat-tat of hail banged off my helmet. The sky dropped white bullets on us.

We placed the bikes under the eves for protection. That's when hail and rain hit harder. As they say, it rained 'cats and dogs' on us. A savage wind blew while marble-sized hail pelted the ground. Several tourists from Maine and Florida drove west to escape the denting of their cars.

We sat for three hours waiting for the downpour to expire. When it did, we returned to the highway where a brilliant rainbow arced halfway up the mountains. We climbed in the late afternoon over a long pass. As it gained altitude, the air grew cooler. At the top, we watched a brilliant sunset. Durango awaited 11 miles away--all downhill from 8,000 feet to 6,500 feet. What a rush of speed, cold and darkness!

Durango is a biking Mecca with a steam engine railroad train. Set into the mountains on the western slope, it's quiet and beautiful.

We found a place to camp in the city park where we cooked up noodle soup and pasta. Even the fabulous Golden Corral dinner didn't taste as good as eating hot soup and pasta at 40 degrees on a park picnic table after racing down a freezing mountain for 11 miles.

Denis wanted to camp in the park. I knew we stood a chance of being evicted by the cops if they discovered us during the night. Oh well, what the heck, we found a place near the bushes as hidden from view as possible.

"Hello in there, Durango police," a man's voice boomed through my nylon at 1:00 in the morning. "You're not allowed to camp in this park."

We were dead meat and would have to pack up and move. Denis started talking to them with his heavy French accent. I remained silent. He explained how we had endured hail, rain, lightning, cold and misery the day before. He explained how we had suffered through freezing weather on our trip from Canada. His voice evoked pity and sadness. He talked to the officers about a grizzly and moose attack that we had lived through. We had been charged by a bison in Yellowstone and were scalded by a geyser. We fell into the frigid waters of Jackson Lake of the Grand Tetons. He told them how a rock nearly crushed us as we slept in a narrow canyon in Utah. He told them that his partner Frosty had an infected foot and had lost his wife in an accident and that this trip was his chance to wash away the pain. When I heard that, I started weeping to give credence to his story. If he kept at it, we might be able to stay. He gave them so much bullshit in his French accent that they were overwhelmed with pity and finally, realizing how deeply we had suffered at the hands of the devil, they apologized for waking him up and asked humbly if we would vacate early in the morning.

As they shuffled away, I whispered, "Brilliant Denis!"

We lucked out on that one. Most cops go by the book in big cities. If it were my brother Howard when he was a cop, he would have kicked me out. Where we had camped out on the ball diamond a day ago in a small city, there was no problem because there were no police. But once in a big city, they nab law breakers like us. They have to, and I don't blame them, but on this night, with Denis' brilliant oratory, we lucked out. Thank goodness they didn't search him for stolen cookies.

Out of Durango on route 550 south. Sunny day. Warm weather. We rode the bike path along the Animas River. Up a long hill we climbed to a Mesa where we headed toward Aztec in New Mexico. Traffic roared past us. No matter as we pedaled on a flat, tailwind assisted highway with farmland of corn, hay and oats. Lots of horses and cows dotted the pastures along the way.

I couldn't get the man out of my mind from the day before who had ridden up to me on his touring bike. He forced me into a conversation. I stood by my bike in front of the City Market jamming food into my panniers.

"Looks like you've got a load," a voice came from behind me.

I turned to see a six foot, brown-haired, 40+ man on his own touring mountain bike. He sported gray sideburns and a few days of stubbled beard. He sported a round face and brown eyes, almost like an older John Belushi, the comedian who died of a drug overdose. His body wasn't quite toned because he looked like he'd been overweight and was still soft around the belly. He looked almost like a grown kid searching for a compliment because he caught a fish or won a stuffed bear at the fair.

"Same might be said for you," I said. "Been ridin' far?"

From the look on his face, I had made his day by asking that question.

"East coast," he said, beaming.

"From your accent," I said, "somewhere in North Carolina."

"Jacksonville," he said. "How could you tell?"

"Lived there as a kid," I said.

"You'd know that accent then," he said.

"Why did you ride east to west?" I asked. "Didn't you hit head winds all the time?"

"It's a long story," he said.

His long story got me caught up in an hour's worth of a man in a life crisis. He had turned 44 and had been a pastor all his life and had never done anything but preach to his flock. Recently, his boss transferred him to another church. He asked for three months off before he had to take up his preaching duties again. His wife agreed to take care of the kids and let him discover himself. Like many men in middle age, he felt the noose of time had begun tightening around his neck.

"I haven't done anything dramatic with my life," he said. "This bike trip has been a turning point. I never knew how much was going on out there before this trip. I only knew my ministry, my congregation and their problems. All I hear about are problems. This country has lost sight of God. I think God directed me in this personal quest so I could serve Him better."

"That's reasonable," I said. "What has been your biggest eye opening experience?"

"What I've missed in life," he said. "I've done every thing by the book. My life's been boring...don't get me wrong. I love my wife and kids but up until this summer, and this great trip, my life's been stale. This trip has given me painful insights."

"Why painful?"

"There are so many choices I didn't know about... never even thought about, or considered," he said.

"Ever hear of the quote by Kate Hepburn?" I asked.

"Yes!" he said, lighting up. "She who follows all the rules all the time misses out on all the fun."

"You got it," I said, surprised that he had heard that quote.

One of his congregation quoted it to him. It was that 'moment' that had spurred him to take the trip. He said God had spoken to him. I, of course, thought it was Kathryn Hepburn. But it didn't matter. He pedaled into a grand adventure. After giving me a 'sermon' on his love of God and how God had directed him, he shoved off- -on his way to San Diego. I thought he wouldn't want to hear my 'take' on God, so I let it be. I didn't want to blow his mind. If I had expounded my 'emerging creative energy' philosophy, he'd probably want to save me! That would have taken another two hours!

I felt genuinely happy for him. He would have a reference point to one epic moment in his life. He could point back to a great physical struggle and heroic accomplishment in the summer at the turn of the century.

So few in this country ever do. Thoreau said it, "Most men live lives of quiet desperation." Their lives slip by quietly--quickly--unspectacularly.

After high school, most people 'fall' into jobs. They rarely go after a job they like because they don't know what they like. If they were lucky enough to go to college, they might find a major that fulfilled their job needs. But, in years since college, I've found many grads working in jobs that have nothing to do with their college majors. After school, most of us fall into 'love', another word for 'lust', and get married. Once the kids come along, our lives for the next 20+ years are locked into child rearing. (or divorce court and visitation rights) That leaves precious little time for ourselves. We fall into the rat race. Life limits our personal time.

As we get tired and bored, as well as fat and out of shape, it's so much easier to click on the TV and watch others live great adventures. We give in to a subtle but destructive life-depression style. It becomes our norm. We can see movies, sports, read books, or see slide shows of others. Before we know it, we're old and can't do anything about it.

I read a book once by Napoleon Hill which gave me a profound idea on life: "There are two ways to look at life: one is that of playing horse while life rides. The other is that of becoming the rider while life plays horse. The choice as to whether one becomes the horse or the rider is the privilege of every person. But this much is certain: if one does not choose to become the rider of life, he or she is sure to become the horse. Life either rides or is ridden. It never stands still."

My dad's early death made sure that I didn't let life slip by or let 'life' ride me. It's why I've been packing it in every year with every ounce of my energies. Amazingly enough, life paths are not a matter of chance, but a matter of choice for humans. Many let the choice be made for them. That's one thing about life...if you don't choose, life will choose for you.

But at my age, with two thirds of my life used up, like water having passed under a bridge, I am acutely aware that I don't have many seasons left. Maybe 20 springs to see the flowers bloom again. Maybe less or a few more, but I'm definitely closer to the grave than the cradle. Yet, I don't feel any urgency because each of my decade birthdays has seen me in some far flung corner of the globe. No mid-life crisis for me! I have been sucking the marrow out of life's bone every year of my existence. I've had fun. I've worked hard. I've played hard. I've danced with my shadow.

But before I know it, my youth will drain from my face and my skin will turn to wrinkles and sag, and the lines will deepen until I too look like Clint Eastwood's craggy face. I remember shaking hands with him at a celebrity ski contest in 1974 in Steamboat Springs, Colorado. He was 45 with deep furrows in his jaw. I was young. He looked old. But the two things that he had that never sagged, or wrinkled or aged were his eyes and attitude.

The fact that time moves more quickly when you age becomes more poignantly apparent with each passing year. A day goes by in a flash and a week vanishes in a wink. A month fades quickly into another and the seasons mesh into the years without notice. If it weren't for my annual Christmas card letter, I wouldn't know what I had done for the past 30 years. It would be a blur.

To give an example of time speeding up as we age, I offer the point of making a child of five stand in the corner for an hour versus a man of 50 standing in a corner for an hour. To the child, one year is one fifth of his life which makes that hour last much longer--because of the child's limited reference points dealing with time. For a man of 50, one year is one fiftieth of his life and therefore, an hour passes more quickly--in a blink if you will.

In my own life, I remember a day at the beach with my parents when I was ten. I had earned a dollar mowing lawns. Every time I got hungry for a 10 cent ice cream sandwich, I bought one. That was one of the longest days of my life because I was deliriously happy from being able to buy what seemed to me an unlimited supply of ice cream sandwiches. To this day, that was the longest, happiest day of my life. In fact, when I get depressed, (Who me? Yeah, me!), I treat myself to a six pack of ice cream sandwiches and it's the cheapest "happy" drug I've ever known. I haven't died from an overdose yet! But what it does tell me is how much our childhoods affect our adult lives. Good and bad.

To get back to my point however, no matter what I do today, whether it's a day at the beach or a day on the slopes skiing, the day is gone in a blink. It's almost like I'm going home from a two day weekend of camping, biking or skiing--moments after I left.

This speeding up of time causes me concern because my life is moving so quickly. But I am given inspiration by a number of 'mentors' who have gone before me in this age thing.

My friend, Sherle Adams, age 80 is a brilliant woman who runs her own business, mentors hundreds of partners, brings energy into a room when she speaks and enthralls thousands with her excitement for life. She has written a best selling book. She's a woman of the 21st century who has been a woman in two centuries. She resides in that rarified air of Susan B. Anthony, Eleanor Roosevelt,

Betty Ford, Margaret Mead and Jane Goodall. I swear that she will live to 110 and still have her running shoes on. If you ever meet her, you won't be able to keep up unless you break into a sub four minute mile!

My dear friend, Duncan Littlefair is 87, yet he attacks each day with gusto unknown to most 20 year olds. He's aware that each day could be his last, yet he revves his mind and charges his body into the day. He gets excited for a country walk. I asked him what he was doing recently. He said, "Nothing! I'm making it an art form. Why does anyone who is retired have to do anything? I'm happy doing nothing." Duncan is one of the 20th century's greatest and most prolific theological minds. He's written books and spoken to and inspired tens of thousands. He is, quite simply, one of the greatest theological minds of the past 3,000 years. If you read his book, "THE GLORY WITHIN YOU," you would know why I say that. He is the one of the men I admire most in the 21st century.

I recall another great Western woman I know named Adeline Helma. She's my Colorado mom. She's in her eighties, but her voice and attitude sound like she's in her twenties. She sparkles with freshness, youth and joy for each day. She loves to dance. The power of her life inspires her kids and friends because she always wakes up on the right side of the bed. She leaps toward the morning sunshine with an attitude of: "What a beautiful day this is going to be." Nothing gets her down, and it's this power of her spirit that gives her kids strength and joy, as well as her friends and anyone she touches. She once gave me a poem by one of her favorite authors, Sam Ullman. In it he writes:

"Youth is not a time of life; it is a state of mind; it is not a matter of rosy cheeks, red lips and supple knees; it is a matter of the will, the quality of the imagination, a vigor of the emotions; it is the freshness of the deep springs of life.

Youth means a temperamental predominance of courage over timidity, of the appetite for adventure over the love of ease. This often exists in a man of 60 more than a boy of 20. Nobody grows old merely by living a number of years. We grow old by deserting our ideals.

Years may wrinkle the skin, but to give up enthusiasm wrinkles the soul. Worry, fear, and self-doubt bows the heart and turns the spirit back to dust.

Whether 60 or 16, there is in every human being's heart the lure of wonder, of unfailing childlike curiosity of what's next, and the joy of the game of living. In the center of your heart and mine there is a wireless station; so long as it receives messages of beauty, hope, cheer and courage, you are young.

When the aerials are down, and your spirit is covered with snows of cynicism and the ice of pessimism, then you have grown old, even at 20. But so long as your aerials are up to catch the optimism, there is hope you may die young at 95."

Thank you Adeline, Duncan, and Sherle.

Chapter 15 — Advance Toward Your Dreams

"If you advance confidently toward your dreams, and endeavor to live the life which you have imagined, you will meet with success unexpected in common hours."

Thoreau

Up ahead, Denis stopped for a drink. Tailwinds made for a pleasant day. The mountains along the route became flat, layered, sedimentary rock with juniper trees growing out of them. As usual, nature amazed me with trees growing out of solid rock. Somehow, roots dig into the rock, creating fissures that hold enough water to keep the tree alive during dry spells.

By the time we reached Aztec, we turned on Route 544 south. The first gold colors of autumn changed with aspens in the high country. A crispness in the air said that old man winter slowly approached. He followed us all the way down from Canada.

We found a campsite off the road in a hilly, sandy motorcycle climbing area. We called the place "Camp

Broken Glass" for all the broken beer bottles and trash from people with guns shooting up the place. But nature fought back by giving us a beautiful sunset with blazing clouds and a crescent moon.

It's a good thing that we will never achieve Star Trek's 'warp speed' because we would find ways to litter and trash the universe.

Next day, we enjoyed a tailwind to Bloomfield where we followed Route 44 to Blanco Station. Tailwinds pushed us along a high desert plateau with barren rock mountains off to the east and west. We traveled on an ancient sea bed with the remaining mountains looking very much like reefs left over from a million years ago.

At Blanco, we cut south on County Road 7900, which led us to "Camp Middle of Nowhere." We traveled deep in Navajo territory. The sunset glowed spectacularly across the horizon as we pitched our tents and ate our dinner sitting among the sagebrush. The sun blazed gold like the fire from a Saturn rocket as it slipped deeper into the earth. Above us, wispy clouds burned yellow and white against a deepening pale blue sky. As soon as the sun set, coyotes howled at the moon--and what a bright, silver and white moon it was. The eastern horizon effervesced into a purple and blue electric sky.

The soup, as always, tasted shall we say, "Exquisite!"

A crow called with the first hint of light in the morning. I stuck my head out to see long shadows working their way across the land as Old Sol made his way into the sky. Just kneeling at my tent opening, I thought about a whole new day. It was mine to do with as I wished. That's the wonder of bicycle touring, I got to be a kid and ride my bicycle—all day. To be a kid while being an adult is a conscious blessing. Why?

Because kids don't think about having the fun they're having! As an adult, not only am I having fun, I'm aware of having fun--and often times on my bike, while touring, I fall into that kid zone where I'm having fun and not even thinking about it. I'm higher than a kite.

We busted our humps over 12 miles of sand and gravel in the morning. Nothing but miles of rolling sagebrush with occasional layers of rocks. In the distance, we saw flat topped mountains. All formed when the area lay beneath an ocean. Because the mountains were stratified, like a multi-layered birthday cake, the junipers grew in horizontal rows to match the striations of rock. It was as if a master gardner had planted each one on purpose.

At White Horse, we hit asphalt again and grabbed some water at an Indian Reservation.

We headed south toward the Continental Divide. It would be our 8th crossing of the Divide since the trip began. Only this time, the terrain had changed. We pedaled in an arid desert. Flat topped mountains prevailed. Scrub juniper dotted the landscape. Dry air sucked the moisture from our bodies. Sand, clay and sagebrush dominated scene--with junipers creating contrast. Many hawks, crows, blackbirds and sparrows flew around us.

By the afternoon, we had covered 50 miles on the rolling highway. We followed a snaking canyon that climbed up and toward the Continental Divide. Soon, we rode along the Divide on Route 509.

At one point, we pulled up a long hill more than four miles to the top, but I never felt it in my legs. No stress. No burn in my thighs. No struggle. My legs had crossed over into that "power zone" where they simply reacted and responded to the needs of the road. My legs were just as happy pedaling on the flats as climbing a mountain. Pedaling a bike was like a bird flapping its wings or a shark flipping its tail or a cheetah racing toward its prey. It was natural. Most of the time, I kept pedaling down a hill from pure habit, even though I was coasting.

On some long inclines, I noticed Denis up ahead. His feet kept dropping down below his panniers. He 'ran' across the land, but never touched down. In effect, he 'flew' above the ground. He mirrored an eagle at the top of a mountain and soared down to the bottom of a valley. When at the bottom, he "flapped" his wings and pedaled back to the top.

I looked down at my own legs. My knees pumped upward toward me and my feet moved down on the power stroke. Unlike a bike racer who "pulls and pushes" through 360 degrees of a pedal stroke, a touring cyclist only presses on the downward stroke of the pedal.

It's never work. It's fun. I'm intrigued why certain people love riding a bike. The answer lies in the sense of flight, of speed while flying, and the rhythm of the rotation of the crank-set that powers them into their flight. After pedaling a few hours, another aspect pops up in the form of endorphins which are produced by the body and are a drug that creates a "happy" high. At the end of many days, I don't want to stop because I'm cruising along on a euphoric bicycle ecstasy. Not only that, but I'm living in the "satori" of the ride--totally absorbed by the riding. It becomes a physical, mental, spiritual euphoria. It feels good to feel so good. I've burst out laughing for no reason at times while riding my bike. Rushes of joy often overwhelm me--and I don't know where come from. I think my body felt so good it made my spirit erupt in laughter which could only be expressed by my face. Where else could my body have expressed the 'great' feeling?

That's the amazing difference between a touring cyclist and a vehicled person. I'm starving to death by 6:00 p.m. from burning 6,000 to 8,000 calories. Dinner offers a grand bouquet. My body is charged with endorphins--and every muscle has played "fun" all day. My spirit is bright and my mind loaded with experiences on a visceral as well as spiritual level. I've been eyeball to eyeball all day with nature. Sight, sound, texture, cold, hot, dry and wet--it's all been there for me. I sleep like a rock.

We made a long pull up an incline along the Continental Divide. Battleship gray skies hung across the mountains in front of us. We stopped to get into our rain suits. Moments later, the sky dumped on us. We splashed through a downpour for a half hour before finding a spot behind an abandoned building.

As luck would have it, three Indians saw us head into the abandoned building and followed us. They walked up, one clearly drunk, and the second seemingly sober.

"Hi," he said, stretching out his hand. "My name is Tim."

"I'm George," the other said.

"We just saw you guys on bikes and wondered what you were doing," Tim said.

Tim offered us a cigarette.

"Smoke?" he said.

"That's okay," Denis said, declining.

We told them about our trip across the country. They were amazed. They thought it was cool what we were doing. George took a whiz in the bushes. He turned around as he zipped up.

"You two ain't queer are you?"

Denis didn't understand the terminology.

"No, we're straight," I said firmly.

"What is queer?" Denis asked me.

"You know, fags," George said.

Denis got out his wallet and showed his wife and kids to the Indians. They seemed satisfied that we weren't two men having a wild affair as we traveled across the country. I wanted to tell them off, but kept quiet.

Moments later, they decided to leave.

"Maybe we'll be back later to party," Tim said.

"We go to sleep early," I said. "We're pretty tired."

We set up our tents and ate dinner. Sure enough, they came back at night fall. I stayed in my tent as Denis talked with them.

George asked, "You guys use travelers checks when you travel?"

"No," Denis said. "We use credit cards."

I reclined in my tent thinking they were sizing us up and what they could steal from us. All sorts of things ran through my mind. This country has gotten so crazy with so many 'nuts' running around that none of us is safe from anything or anyone anymore.

After five minutes, they decided to leave.

I popped out of my tent clearly worried.

"If those guys get drunk and decide to come back tonight," I said. "We could be in for some trouble."

"I don't think they will bother us," Denis said.

"No telling what a couple of drunks might do, Denis," I warned. "We will have to keep one eye open all night."

Denis spent the next half hour erecting a barricade of barbed wire and scrap iron from the abandoned building. He set it up over the cattle guard and driveway that led into our compound. After Denis finished, it looked like something right out of a "ROAD WARRIORS" movie with Mel Gibson. They would have to make noise getting through the wire and metal gate.

"At least this way, if they come in the night," Denis said. "We'll hear them crash their car into the wire fence."

From that moment, we made our escape plans. We would hear the noise and quickly leave our tents for the deep grasses where we couldn't be found. They might steal our gear, but they wouldn't be able to see us to kill us.

I dropped back thinking about how I would get out of my tent and hide if I heard them. No telling what could happen if I stayed to be a victim. I didn't want to be a news headline in the local paper.

The whole scene reminded me of a tour from coast-to-coast that I took in 1984 when I was in Alabama on the last leg of my cross continent journey. A guy stopped me in a pickup truck and offered to take me to meet his wife and kids, plus I was welcome to a shower and dinner.

"I'd love to have you meet my wife," he said. "She's a former Playboy Bunny."

"Wow, that's great," I said, wondering why he had made such a ridiculous statement about his wife.

"She bakes a great pecan pie," he said.

As I stood there, it didn't feel right. In the past, I had been stopped by dozens of people who had invited me into their homes. I had been wined and dined by millionaires. Bank presidents wanted to hear my story.

Doctors and their wives cooked me five course dinners. An oil man in Texas gave me the keys to his cottage, sailboat, jet skis, speed boat and wind surfers. John Brown and I lived in a mansion for three days.

I'll never forget the man named Spencer in Graham, Texas. "I just wanna' show you boys a little Texas hospitality," he drawled.

Filthy rich and bored to death, Spencer wished he was riding with us. But instead, he wanted to hear our story.

But this guy standing in front of me made me feel uneasy. Why would you tell any stranger that you had a Playboy Bunny for a wife?

"Guess I'll get on down the road," I said.

"Sure now?" he said.

"Yeah," I said. "I need to make some miles before the sunset."

Before he said anything further, I shoved off.

"Thanks and have a good evening," I said with a nod.

A month later back home, my brother, who lived across the street from me at the time, got a phone call from a sheriff in Alabama asking if Frosty Wooldridge was his brother.

"Sure is," Howard said.

"Well son," the sheriff drawled. "We think we have his body....he was shot and left dead on the road and we've finally tracked him to your home phone."

"Can't be my brother," Howard said. "I just spoke with him ten minutes ago."

Howard learned from the sheriff that a bicyclist had been shot and his body dumped along side the road where I had traveled. The guy looked like me and had a mustache and was riding across country. The reason they found out my name was that I had stopped at a convenience store and had gotten into a conversation with the local man who rode bikes and he had read a bunch of my stories from the early 80s on Alaska. So, when the sheriff asked if he knew anything, the local man told him about the magazine and that I was a writer for them. So, they called and got my brother's phone number. That's when they called Howard up and said they thought they had his dead brother at their morgue.

Good thing I wasn't too keen on seeing that guy's Playboy Bunny wife! Probably saved my life.

Nonetheless, we camped out in the middle of nowhere and if a band of drunks came by in the dark of night, we'd be in trouble. That night, I looked like Popeye the Sailor Man with one eye open and an ear to the air. At one point in the night, an animal made a noise outside my tent which bolted me awake.

Scared the daylights out of me!

CHAPTER 16 — ONE PERSON MAKES A DIFFERENCE

"One final paragraph of advice: Do not burn yourselves out. Save the other half of yourselves and your lives for pleasure and adventure. It is not enough to fight for the land; it is even more important to enjoy it. While you can. While it's still here. While you're here. So get out there and hunt and fish and mess around with your friends, ramble out yonder and explore the forests, encounter the grizzly, climb the mountains, bag the peaks, run the rivers, breathe deep of that yet sweet and lucid air, sit quietly for a while and contemplate the precious stillness, that lovely, mysterious and awesome space. Enjoy yourselves, keep your brain in your head and your head firmly attached to the body--the body active and alive, and I promise you this much: I promise you this one sweet victory over your enemies, over those desk bound people with their hearts in a safe deposit box and their eyes hypnotized by desk top calculators. I promise you this: you will out live the bastards."

Edward Abbey
Desert Solitaire
Monkey Wrench Gang

Morning sunrise broke over the peaks! We lived!

A clear sky to the west promised a great cycling day. I tore down the barricade and pedaled out to the highway. We rode a one percent downhill grade for miles—with a tail wind.

Route 605 took us into Route 66 toward Grants. Yes, we rode historic Route 66 for more than ten miles. It was a little more than interesting to me because my mom had packed the 53 Chevy station wagon 45 years ago and drove Route 66 with four kids out to San Diego. We hopped a plane and flew to Hawaii to be with our dad who was stationed at the Marine base in Hawaii. My daddy was a Marine and I was proud to wear a T-shirt proclaiming it. I was eight.

More intriguing was the fact that mom had stopped at a Dairy Freeze on Route 66 and bought us all a five cent cone. The man who owned it was a comedian who loved to entertain. He squirted a yellow string of 'mustard' out of a hot dog and gave out hamburgers that squeaked. By sheer accident, I stopped by his place 44 years later—and he was still there! He didn't remember me, but I remembered him. He is still at it—making kids smile with his bag of tricks. He must have entertained hundreds of thousands of kids for five decades. I was so astounded I could hardly contain myself.

You know, there are some people that come into our lives for one brief, shining moment. They touch us with what is good in this world. They make us laugh or cry with joy, and never ask a penny. They tell us stories or volunteer for a meaningful project in their community. They never receive a hero's welcome or hear proclamations by dignitaries of their many accomplishments. Only their families know of their good deeds. Even though they have had just as challenging a time in their own journey, they make our journey a bit lighter, more fun and certainly more enjoyable. There is an old statement in the Good Book that I find to be more profoundly true with each passing year: "It is better to give than receive." The ice cream man made that his lifelong gift to the world.

A friend of mine, Norm Waldman, exemplifies this precious shared energy. At 76, he says he is "The Spirit of 76." Every time I see him, he's got that sparkle in his eye and a ready smile.

"How you doin' Norm?" I ask.

"Best day yet!" he always replies.

He doesn't have an ice cream stand but the 'ice cream cones' that he gives to everyone he touches are just as tasty, fun and nourishing--because Norm nourishes peoples' souls. He gives their spirits a lift. He proves daily that it is better to give than receive.

I wonder if the magic of that statement is the reason those individuals are so happy?!

We pedaled into Grants and stopped for food supplies. Once again Condor creaked with the added weight. I felt his sluggishness when fully loaded with water and three days of food. In South America, I carried an extra free wheel, chain, rear derailleur, two tubes and two spare tires. That added an extra ten pounds at all times. At one stretch, I loaded seven days of food onto my bike. It was like riding a pack mule. Condor never complained, and my legs were so strong they didn't either. When I look back, that was my greatest adventure. I'd ride South America again in a blink.

We pedaled further east until we reached a minor black road heading south into the mountains. I had no idea of what we were heading into. As we pedaled over a hill, we rode along a towering red and tan sandstone line of cliffs. They intimidated us by their 300 foot boldness. Big block boulders had broken off in several places to crash near the road. To our right, an unbroken line of black lava appeared along the roadway. It was frozen in place but looked as if it were flowing southward. In places it looked like thick black pancake batter that had piled up in circular layers. Trees and scrubs grew out of it in the cracks.

I looked at the map. We rode through the Valley of Fires. A volcano 1500 years ago now known as Mount Taylor exploded and sent lava 44 miles along the valley floor. It's still there and in many places, so toxic to plants, nothing grows on it. It measured five miles wide and 160 feet thick in places. It remained perfectly preserved as if a slow motion movie had stopped.

We looked off into the distance to the west to see a huge gray squall line headed toward us. It measured three miles wide and looked like one of those disaster movies coming at us.

"Let's beat it," I yelled.

"Pedal hard!" Denis said.

If we could make three miles in 15 minutes, we could make the blue sky on the outside of the squall line. We bent down on our aero bars, (race bars to give us a low profile and point us over the bars), and kicked it into high gear. Like two little kids who had made a candy bar bet on who could get to the corner first--we laughed and yelled as we hammered the pedals. Like tiny ants avoiding the on-rushing death of a tidal wave by racing to high ground, we pushed our steeds as fast as our legs pumped. The squall kept coming and we kept racing to beat it.

After ten minutes we were three-quarters past it, but it closed fast. Man and machine versus nature's fury. We kept the pace. Raindrops sprinkled on us at first. Denis zoomed ahead, but I fell behind. The sprinkles became a torrent and the torrent became a downpour. I struggled, but kept going. I was almost ahead of it, when a wall of water dropped out of the sky, like someone pouring a bucket of water onto a fire. I looked like a cat that had just gotten pulled out of a tub of water. Another mile riding in the rain brought me to the El Malpais National Monument visitor center. I pulled under an overhang to get out of the rain.

"You're wet," Denis said. "No drops touched me."

"You're such a Frenchman," I said.

We toured the center. Zuni, Laguna, Acoma, and Navajo lived on the land for 10,000 years. They built villages and grew crops. For centuries, they traded and fought one another. Their ways came to a halt when the white man invaded them.

El Malpais means "badlands" in Spanish. The heat in the summer will kill you and the cold in the winter will freeze you. Water is a scarce resource. The 44 miles of lava flow offers stunning natural beauty. It's primal, pristine, weird and inviting. Touring the center gave us an appreciation for the people who once lived there. Survival was their daily struggle.

So few of us today think about survival any more. We can eat food from the cabinet or fridge at our whim-- and order pizza or go out to dinner at a fancy restaurant. A click of the switch gives cool or warm air.   A shower each day is automatic. Those people fought off disease, wolves, bears, harsh weather, human enemies and pretty much lived at the mercy of the elements. They didn't have ski vacations, trips to Europe, evenings at the movies, or Christmas gifts. No one read or wore sunglasses or eyeglasses. Makeup? Forget it. A mirror was unknown to them. They didn't have TV, taxes, time, wheels or birthdays.   There was no such thing as a calendar or wristwatch. There were no jails, police or judges. No one was richer or poorer. They lived a profoundly different life than we know today.

The rain stopped. Once again, we cranked southward toward a collection of mountains that could be described as a group of large waves heading into a beach. A dark sky provided the mist. Their tan colors resembled white foamy crests. We pedaled alongside them. They towered 300 feet above us with black lava flows bending and weaving off to our right.

In a half-hour we arrived at La Ventanna, New Mexico's largest natural arch. We walked up to it from a small trail. It was like walking under the Golden Gate Bridge--enormous, elegant, and sublime.

As we stood under it, the sky rushed toward us over the high sandstone cliffs five hundred feet above us. Rain fell as mist followed by a tidal wave monsoon and drenched us within seconds. The wind howled like a pack of hungry wolves. It was a 'bad hair' day.

I jumped under a pinion tree. As I stood there, rain splashed on my head, dripped on my feet, and ran down my arms and legs. A small river formed on the path and quickly rushed down the hillside. I braved it like an antelope or coyote standing in the rain. The rain soaked and chilled me. I knew what an animal experienced.

After the initial deluge, we mounted the bikes, and pedaled off in a drizzle. To the right, black lava fields folded onto each other like a thick chocolate cake batter being poured into a pan. On our left, vertical sandstone/ red walls rose into the sky. It wasn't long before we found a camping spot under a large sandstone wall.

The rain stopped for a half-hour. We commenced pitching our tents when Denis yelled, "Look, the rain is coming."

"Sure is," I said as I looked up to see a sheet of rain advancing on us at high speed.

We tossed gear into the tents, but we weren't fast enough. It roared in and hit us with another blast of water.

I sat in the tent with my miner's lamp lighting the notebook while the rhythmic splatter of heavy rain beat its own music onto my little wilderness dwelling. Constant splatter of each raindrop that made the music. Sometimes, it let up and drizzled, but again came in like violins in a symphony. In the distance, thunder rattled the sky and the lightning flashed through my tent. I curled into my sleeping bag atop my air mattress--and, although the world around me was wet--I stayed dry.

Camp Grenada!

CHAPTER 17 — LIVE OR DIE AT NATURE'S WHIM

"Let's just wander here and there like leaves floating in the autumn air and look at common little things-- stones on the beach flowers turning into berries-- from the winds we'll catch a bit of that wondrous feeling that comes not from seeing but from being a part of nature."

Gwen Frostic

Lying in the tent, I woke up thinking about John Brown. Half way across the world in Australia, he'll wake up today with only one thought on his mind, and that is to beat the disease that is trying to kill him. He's probably sick to his stomach with chemotherapy. From what I've heard, the cure makes you feel like you wish you were dead. As I ruminated in my sleeping bag--warm and secure in my world-- thousands of miles away, he waged a titanic struggle to live.

Funny thing about health and living for so many people. They take it for granted. Every time I see a smoker, I wonder what is going on in his or her mind.

What possesses someone to invite cancer or emphysema into their bodies? Why do millions of beer and liquor drinkers try to pickle their livers? Why do they want to cut their lives short? This nation includes 100 million fat people who know obesity will severely affect their lives, yet they continue over-eating. They keep eating that which is sure to cause an early death, or make them miserable while living with degenerative diseases such as bad knees, diabetes, hardened arteries, etc.

While back at that Golden Corral where Denis and I ate ourselves sick, I watched one cowboy with a tan ten-gallon hat and a large rodeo belt buckle on his jeans. He limped, from what looked like a bad hip, into the restaurant. His colorful cowboy shirt ballooned out like an ocean wave trying to roll over his belt. He was 90 pounds over weight with a face that looked like Garfield the Cat after he'd eaten 50 mice. He sat down with his two small children and wife. When the waitress gave them their plates, he skipped the salad bar and headed straight for the beef, pork, sausages and gravy. While Denis and I devoured the fruit, salad and veggie bars, that guy 'inhaled' half a cow and a few pigs.

Later, he finished by shoveling half the dessert bar onto his plate. I couldn't help feeling sorry for his kids. They might not have their father at their high school graduations. He would not be proud of them in their sports or academic pursuits--because his overwhelming chances for an early death were acute.

Back at camp, as I looked at my tent ceiling, I tried to figure out why John suffered cancer? He followed a life of fit, trim, health and nutrition consciousness. He exposed himself to lots of sun from living on the beach all his life, but his was lymphoma cancer. Maybe too much sun over 50 years added up to his type of cancer. Who knows?

Whatever the case, he's in a battle for his life.

I remember hearing when Walter Peyton, one of the greatest NFL running backs to ever set foot on a football field, contracted a rare liver disease at age 45. Soon after, he contracted cancer. He knew he would die within months. He said he was scared. He prayed. He cried. What did he do as he woke up each day KNOWING life escaped him too early? He conquered behemoths on the gridiron, but got taken out by tiny viruses. Was it fair?

There is nothing fair on this planet. There's only hope, luck of birthplace, and reasonable action to give each of us a better chance for living to old age. Those who don't enjoy that 'luck' or birthplace, simply suffer a miserable life and/or early death from disease or starvation.

As a cardiac catheterization technician 25 years ago, I saw people struggling for their lives and wishing to God they hadn't smoked or eaten such poor diets. Most of them were in their mid to late forties and early fifties. They STILL possessed a great desire to live, but their actions had piled up against them for too many years and they had damaged their bodies beyond repair.

They knew they were going to die.

As a young hospital technician, I watched people die on the operating table. I heard wails, screams and cries from loved ones. I watched lives shortened before their time. It was an incomplete life, like being arrested against your will and being taken out of your favorite movie-- never seeing the ending. Never tasting or enjoying the whole thing!

For those who keep over-eating, drinking or smoking, they too, one day, too soon, may meet their maker. Me? I will too, but I'm going to try to make it as late a death as possible. I like what the late comedian George Burns said, "It's the first 100 years that's easy."

After having contemplated John's battle with cancer, I poked my head out to greet the morning. The sky broke blue above me and a few clouds shrouded the peaks south of us, but it sparkled crystal clear to the horizon. A magpie hopped across the front of my tent. He must have been looking for bugs. Glad I'm not a bird. One bug down my throat was enough in my lifetime. We packed our gear wet and ate breakfast. Denis was slow getting his packs loaded so I took off. Within several miles, I passed the lava falls area where lava had cascaded over some high ground and dropped like a waterfall, only frozen in place for 1500 years.

After another ten miles, the lava field came to a stop along the highway. Before me was 40 miles of open, endless prairie. A chain of craters dotted the flat landscape where I pedaled. A 25-mile per hour head wind distressed me. When added to my 10-mph speed, it exceeded a 35 mile per hour head wind that relentlessly pushed against me for the next five hours. I bulldozed into it with steadfast determination. Soon, I became like a mule...mile after mile, head down, pedaling strong, determined in my journey.

The one thing about a head wind -- you have two choices--keep going or give up. It's discouraging and can break a person's resolve. At nature's whim by adding another twenty miles per hour of head winds, I would be busted. My efforts would fail trying to move forward.

For me, it's an example, however slight--how fragile, how vulnerable humans are in the face of nature. Mother Nature can suck us in and spit us out in the blink of an eye. Hurricane Floyd ripped up the coast of the USA in 1999 and displaced 2.5 people and eight billion dollars in damage. In 2005, a hurricane named Katrina brought death and destruction beyond anyone's imagination. It could not have cared a twit whether anyone of them lived or died. In Africa, 11 million humans perished in the past ten years of AIDS--and millions more are expected to die. Yet, Africa's population is one of the fastest growing in the world having doubled to 767 million since 1960. According to the World Health Organization, 40,000 children under the age of 10 die of starvation or related diseases each day. All totaled, eight million people die from starvation annually worldwide.

Makes me think that nature is on the side of the viruses and famine, but then, still decides to warrant millions more human babies. It's hard to figure.

At the same time, John Brown fights for his life. After calling home a few nights ago, I found out that a friend in my dance club, Paula, came down with ovarian cancer. She's a great dancer and I've danced with her over the years. She's an incredibly lovely lady and she married a wonderful man. I was flabbergasted. Everyone was praying for her, but in reality, those prayers fall on the deaf ears of the universe. Like John, she may live, or she may die--depending on the luck of the draw.

It's most disconcerting to know that we humans mean so little to the forces of nature. Or is it? Maybe it's better to know it and accept it. And, get on with the business of living. If we die too soon, it was our unlucky star. It's all so capricious.

Have you ever wondered what you would be doing if you only had a year to live? Think about it. My question to you is: why aren't you doing it now? What are you waiting for?

Indeed, for many, it is a cruel, heartless world. For me, pedaling into a nasty head wind, it might be grueling for five hours, but I'm thankful just to be healthy enough to do it. A lot of people wonder why I'm so positive and high all the time and it seems obvious--just to be healthy, with a roof over my head and food to eat is enough to cheer about. The rest is gravy. Sometimes, I feel like getting down on my knees and crying in thanks for being healthy. Come on John and Paula--I send you my energy. We will ride and dance again.

At Route 36, I turned south toward Macado. The wind blew down on me from the side. Tolerable. Denis caught up and we pedaled together. Macado was a junk town with the only nice building being the post office. We grabbed some water and turned on Route 32 into the Apache National Forest where we pedaled for six miles until we stopped in some juniper trees to camp beside the road.

It was a beautiful windy day. I'll take head winds over disease, war and famine.

A spectacular purple sunrise broke over the mountains in the morning. A spaceship saucer-cloud glowed with light from behind. Dew covered the tents and our constant friends the mosquitoes kept us busy swatting away their pesky advances. We gobbled oatmeal, bananas and bread for breakfast.

Within 20 miles, the road had climbed to 7,000 feet. A dense covering of trees dotted golden grasses that waved in the breeze. We turned south on Route 12 at Apache Creek. A small ram shackled grocery with a porch and a gas pump was the only sign of humanity. Two old men sat swatting flies while talking in Spanish. They appeared happy doing nothing because they had nothing to do. We asked them for water and they pointed. No sense in wasting energy on a hot day.

The road followed a dry river valley until it reached Reserve Village where we loaded up on more water. From there we turned south on 180 toward Silver City.

Pine trees covered 11,000 foot mountains. Their deep green profiled against a pale blue sky. Rocky dry stream beds seemed the norm. Brown grasses and wilted sunflowers lined the road as we climbed higher. At the top of the serpentine road, we reached Saniz Pass at 6,436 feet. The air turned cool.

Soon, we rushed downward, driven by our gravity motors--into a wide valley with a muddy river and cacti growing everywhere. Spinny, prickly, spears--all cactus plants. Often, gorgeous red flowers with yellow centers beckoned our eyes.

At Greenwood, we stopped at a campground and a $3.00 shower. Once again, the road dust, grime, dried salt and stinky clothes washed away in the warm water. You probably don't want to hear that olfactory episode again! Suffice to say, I smelled like an Aqua Velva Man afterwards.

I talked to a silver haired man from Prescott, Arizona who was enthralled that anyone would ride a bike for several thousand miles. He said he wished he could do it or would have done it as a younger man. When he found out that he was only two years older than me, he was a bit astounded.

Back at camp, Denis cooked dinner. Later, I kept thinking about Paula and John's cancers. I wondered about my own emotions and worries. Does anyone have a peaceful life today? It seems that life has so many crushing problems with jobs, family, money, health and relationships. It amazes me anyone keeps their head above water. It's little wonder more people don't escape to drugs, booze and food. Enough do!

I'll try to keep a balance and my life accented on the positive. As I sit at this picnic table, a brilliant full moon crests the mountains to the east. I've watched it each night as it started from crescent to quarter to half to three quarter to this magical silver orb above me. Right now, it's rising over the rocks...hanging elegantly in the sky like one of those glowing globes in a James Bond movie. It is a silver white orb with a face--the old man in the moon--the one who inspired songs and love for centuries. I love those songs: "By the light...of the silvery moon," and another, "Moon river, wider than a mile, I'm crossing you in style someday....you dream maker, you heart breaker...."

Have you ever kissed by the light of a full moon? Great isn't it! If you haven't, grab your lover and get out there. It's magical!

The one thing about being on a bicycle adventure is that it allows anyone closer connections with the rhythms of nature. I notice the flight of birds every day and the owl's hoot at night. The crow calls each morning or a rooster on a farm gives his greeting to the morning, "Cock ah doodle dooo!" The wind plays in my face and the stillness of the evening enchants my spirit. Sometimes when I walk at dusk, it's so quiet, I can hear my clothes moving on my body. While I walk, the rushing waters of a stream might inspire me or calm me. A storm moving in may excite me. The campfire warms my body as well as calms my mind. To sit on the eastern edge of a lake at sunset and watch that golden line of light reach across the waters causes a spiritual glow in my heart. To sit with my friend Denis and know all is right with our world—well—Gwen Frostic was right, "...that wondrous feeling does not come from seeing nature, but from being a part of nature."

CHAPTER 18 — SPOKES ROLLING DOWN HILL

"As you think, you travel; and as you love, you attract. You are today where your thoughts have brought you; you will be tomorrow where your thoughts take you. You can not escape the result of your thoughts, but you can endure and learn....you will realize the vision (not the idle wish) of your heart, be it base or beautiful...for you will always gravitate toward that which you, secretly most love. Whatever your present environment may be, you will fall, remain or rise with your thoughts, your vision, your ideal. You will become as small as your controlling desire; as great as your dominant aspiration."

James Allen

We crossed the Continental Divide (6,326 feet) for the last time on the adventure. The day saw us cranking up and down hills, ever climbing, coasting downward and up again. We pedaled past flowers and cacti. The mountains diminished slowly into hills.

Heat made us suck down water as we dripped it out of our skin on every climb. We rolled along on a straight, flat highway and noticed the rivers ran dry. Big Dog Creek, Little Dry Creek, Empty River, Rock Creek, Sand Creek--all of them had no water.

Near the end of the day, we stopped for a water break when an old man drove up his driveway on a 40 year old Ford Tractor. We started talking and the conversation evolved into thoughts about living and dying. He said he admired Dr. Kervorkian.

"If my life isn't worth living'," he said. "I should have the right to end it."

"You're not wrong there," I said. "Have you ever heard of the movie Soylent Green?"

"Sure have," he said. "Edward G. Robinson and Charlton Heston...."

He described the part where the world was overpopulated to such an extent that humans had to eat dead humans as food. He liked it where Robinson came to the moment where his life was ending from being so old that he couldn't enjoy it any more. During that futuristic time, Robinson visited a dying chamber where he sat down in an easy chair with a movie screen in front of him. He picked his favorite music and a movie of wilderness places where deer came down to a lake to drink. A blue sky profiled with mountains was highlighted with birds winging across the water. Unseen engineers allowed Robinson an hour of beauty, music and nature. He drank a Hemlock concoction and fell asleep peacefully.

Not all life ends so pleasantly for most humans. Few enjoy the choice or die in their sleep. On a tour through the Sierra Madres of California in 1989, I rode up the 49er Trail with my friend Doug. We had eaten lunch under a shady tree alongside the road. We were ready to go when I held us up for another minute because I had to take a bathroom break. Back on the road, we cranked up a hill with sweat dripping from our bodies. Not five minutes later, we saw a bicyclist coming the other way as we rolled into the valley. At the bottom, he coasted to a stop. Doug and I slowed down to greet him.

I looked at the bike rider when I noticed he carried a black puppy on a platform on his rear rack. I smiled, "What a nice...." I began to say. Before I could finish my sentence, the puppy bounded off the platform and ran across the pavement toward us. I heard a vehicle coming, but before the driver or anyone could bat an eyelash, the puppy yelped in a death cry after being crushed by two sets of wheels from a pickup truck going 60 miles per hour.

From a happy disposition with blue sky and sunshine overhead, pained jerked me into bewilderment. My first thought was for the fellow across the road that had seen his puppy crushed to death before his eyes. Blood gushed from the dog's body.

"Oh no," I said in a withered voice.

It shocked my senses from a lovely day to a terrible moment that happened with no rhyme or reason. Only that moment. Had we eaten lunch for 30 seconds longer, or had I waited to relieve myself, the exact meeting of that fellow bicyclist would have saved the puppy. I grew sick with the scene in front of me.

The rider got off this bike. He walked across the road, picked up the dog and walked up to us.

"I'm so sorry," I said with grief in my voice.

"Nothing you could do," he said. "It wasn't anyone's fault."

The driver stopped and ran back, "I'm sorry," he said. "I couldn't stop."

"There's nothing you could have done, sir," the bicyclist said. "Thanks for stopping."

"I'm sorry son," the driver said as he walked away.

"I'm so sorry," I repeated. "Is there anything I can do?"

"No," he said. "I need to take Sierra for a walk in the woods."

As he carried the pup away toward the trees, I stood there, my heart crushed with pain. He had lost a special friend; one he had run through the high country with; one who had sat by campfires with him.

A half-hour passed before I walked up to where he buried Sierra. I introduced myself. His name was Bob and he began crying. I embraced him. His pain moved into me. I wept with tears running down my face onto his shirt, soaking a small circle into it. I held him tight. He talked with his face on my shoulders, sniffling through his nose, convulsing with gasps of air. Minutes later, we picked up rocks and finished covering Sierra's body. Bob and I walked back toward the road. Bob didn't look back, but his whole being was torn. I sensed the anguish ripping at his foundations.

"I don't understand why this happened," he said.

Doug nor I said anything. What could we say? What could we do?

Nothing!

Bob decided to continue south. He wanted to figure out why this had happened. I gave him one last hug. Doug did too. Bob walked across the road, picked up his bike and rode off carrying more pain than his panniers could handle.

"Do you know only one car has ridden by us in the last 30 minutes?" Doug said.

"This blows me away."

"Eat dessert first."

"What?"

"I read it on one of those climber's T-shirts in Yosemite, it said, 'Eat dessert first, life is uncertain.'"

"No kidding," I said. "Let's get going."

I pulled my bike from the gravel shoulder. I grasped the bars with both hands. Looking down, I slipped my right foot into the pedal strap. I pressed hard. The wheels gleamed as they advanced. For the first time in my life, I noticed the spokes go forward and backward simultaneously. They rotate up as well as down while the bike travels along the road. There's no power stroke for the spokes. They merely carry the load placed on them. On the end of the spokes, the wheel rolls around. Just like this planet revolves in space. No reason--other than that's the way it is. I don't know why Sierra died. No reason. I fell in behind Doug, watching his freewheel spin forward, looking at his derailleur as it dropped the chain into lower gears when we began climbing out of the valley. For the rest of the day, I watched his spinning back wheel.

Sitting in the tent that night, the light had faded and the last bird had ruffled its feathers in silence. The mountain air was hushed and my candle flame flickered quietly. I shall never forget that day, or its message--eat dessert first, for life is uncertain. Take it all in daily--joy and sorrow, good times and bad, confidence and uncertainty, smiles and tears, love and heart break--because this is the best moment of life, present living. At no time are any of us immune to misfortune no matter what our situation in life.

I have eaten dessert first--most of my life, but that night, I wasn't hungry. The one thing I learned that day was that everything has an ending. Make the most of the game before it ends. Make the most of your life before it vanishes into eternity.

After our talk on death and Kervorkian, the tractor man talked about the traffic and life in general. Yet he was happy because he worked the land and enjoyed his solitude. We rode off when he slipped his tractor into gear and made his way back down the dirt road to his barn.

A few miles out of Silver City, we crossed the Continental Divide again and stopped at a Golden Corral. Yes, we stuffed ourselves sick. Some kids never learn.

After dinner, we met a college student who had ridden the Divide with a trailer attached to his bike called a "Bob." He was going to touch the border and ride back to Iowa.

An hour later, we found a field and pitched our tents.

Next day, rolling toward the border, we caught high gear on a hot, sunny morning. Rock mountains lined our path with cacti everywhere along the road. It was sun baked desert hell. The sun cooked everyone like a broiled chicken. There was no relief. From the first hour it popped over the horizon, until it boiled like a caldron into the desert sand in the west--the sun burned, baked and fried everything in that inferno-like land.

It was only 95 degrees that day because it was nearly October. A month previous and we would have been toasted as we pedaled. Even with our 7,000 to 4,000 foot loss of altitude, it was hot. We rolled along at 20 miles per hour and made 50 miles to Deming in three hours. We flew along like two F-16 Tomcat jet fighters. Along the highway, cacti with spikes ready to defend themselves from intruders, dotted desert sands. In the distance on our left and right, sand devils swirled dust into the air. In front, a flotilla of dry, tan, rock mountains rose out of the desert like a fleet of war ships on their last mission.

Heat! It beat down on man, beast and bicycle. The road turned into a dream-like mirage as we pedaled along the black asphalt. Cars emerged from it and passed us. A road runner, only the second one of my life, jumped out of the bushes and scrambled back in as quickly when he saw us coming.

Water was the prime directive for the day's ride. Denis complained, "My water bottle is hot and the water is too hot."

"Like my old drill sergeant said, "If you don't like warm water in the desert, try drinking sand."

"What other wisdom did he give?" Denis asked.

"Well," I said. "We were having a barracks inspection on a Saturday when he asked if we were getting enough sleep."

Everyone yelled, "Yes sergeant!"

Like a damned fool, I yelled. "No sergeant!"

"Who said that?" he snapped.

"I did," I said. "We're only getting three and one-half hours sleep per night and it's not enough to become a good soldier."

"How much sleep do you need cadet?" he asked, standing eyeball to eyeball to me with his teeth gnashed and his fists balled up into white knuckles.

I could see the red lines running through his eyeballs. He was none too happy with me.

"Six hours per night, sir," I said, thinking the Army really cared about anyone's comfort levels.

"To catch up," he snarled, "you're confined to your bunk for the weekend...that means the shitter and ten minutes for chow only...Got it cadet?"

"Yes sergeant!" I said, withering under his Gestapo tactics.

It was the last time I ever stood up for right or truth, justice and the American Way in the U.S. Army.

Denis laughed.

We had talked a lot about our lives on the tour. We'd be pedaling along when someone popped up with a topic. We covered women, politics, race, continents, things we'd done, people we'd remembered--all about something or nothing as we shared the road.

The highway grew hotter and the air felt like someone had shoved a hair dryer into our faces and turned it up to high. The heat sucked moisture out of our pores.

We persevered because we were on a bicycle adventure. I always give myself thoughts of a reward when I make the next destination. A half gallon of cold orange juice is my biggest reward. I remember once in Bolivia where we had no food or human contact for six days. We scrapped the bottom of the food bags with rice and oatmeal. I promised myself a treat of canned peaches when we hit the next town. We passed a military check point where a colonel marched out to see who could be crazy enough to ford all those rivers and climb to 15,500 feet in the Andes on bicycles. He shook our hands.

At the first vendor, I saw ten cans of peaches. I bought two. To this day, the first can was the best tasting and most deliciously flavorful, sweetest peaches in the world. The second can caused me delirious ecstasy. No peaches before or since have risen to the level of those two cans of peaches.

At Deming, we felt like we rode off the end of the earth. We faced flat, dry desert and no mountains. A black strip of asphalt stretched to the horizon. Mexico-- 34 miles away. We tanked up on more water and headed down the road under a scorching, blistering sun. No mercy. Cruel. Relentless.

Had we made that area five weeks ago, we'd be a couple of fried chili peppers. We would have needed three gallons of water to go from town to town. In Columbus, only three miles from the border, we drank a half gallon of orange juice. It ran down my throat with pure pleasure.

Under a blazing sun, we remounted the bikes and headed the last few miles to Mexico.

Mexico, that sprawling, sun baked desert land, holds 104 million people. The border patrol passed us a dozen times on our way down from Deming. They try to catch the estimated three million illegals that cross every year, but it's useless as the politics and money are in someone else's hands. We, as a country, keep fooling ourselves at our own expense at letting in millions of illiterate people who have no vested stake in our country. We could stop it by passing prohibitive/severe laws for anyone employing them, but we don't so we pay as our country becomes inundated with them. On the human level, I can't blame them, because they are living in wretched conditions in most Third World countries. I'd try myself.

But even as we take in a million legally and another three million illegally, another 77 million are born into mass poverty annually around the globe. We can't save them all, but we can destroy our own country. It's a matter of population problems. The USA with 300 million people is overpopulated because one American uses 10 to 30 times more raw resources than a Third World person.   By doing the math, you can see that the USA has the worst overpopulation problem in the world. At our current rate of growth, we will add 100 million people by 2040. Name one advantage to adding 100 million people to the United States in three short decades.   One day in this century, it's going to rear its ugly head and bite all of us.

At the border we took pictures and toasted John Brown. We wished him good health and victory over cancer. I couldn't help hoping that one day in the future, he too would ride this great Continental Divide route.

There we stood, hands raised in triumph in front of the sign that read, "Welcome to Mexico."

We had succeeded in a monumental undertaking--2400 miles, nine crossings of the Continental Divide, thousands of pedal strokes, five national parks, two national monuments, the Lewis and Clark Expedition Center, the Mountain Man Museum, Livingston Train Museum, spectacular sunrises and sunsets, hundreds of people and miles of smiles.

We pedaled back to Poncho Villa State Park three miles from the border. The entire park featured a giant cactus garden.

As I sat there with my candle lantern flickering, a thousand crickets chirped their ancient songs. It never changes. It's a symphony of night music. Above, a clear black sky hung motionless above with an orange glow on the western horizon. A cool breeze kept mosquitoes away. I sat in a cactus garden in the middle of the desert. The rising full moon lit the sky and created shadows across the land. Condor, my bike, stood quietly near my tent, motionless, but ready. I knew he was only a piece of steel and rubber, but he was my steed--the one I chased after windmills with, and fought dragons. How could a warrior be without his trusty steed? For me, Condor was my winged horse, my magic ride, my velvet carpet. He carried me to great heights in my life both physically and spiritually.

Across from me, Denis wrote in his own journal. He is a kind, gentle man. This trip underscored our friendship of 19 years. His thoughts were of Christian and his children Florence and Alexis. Soon, he would be with them. What an honor to ride with Denis after all these years. Within a week, we will go back to our routine lives.

But for one shinning moment, across North America, we bicycled the Continental Divide. We labored up mountain passes, battled vicious head winds and rode in cold rains. No matter what the challenge, we kept pedaling our way over mountains and plains. We met people and raced a few dogs. We got honked at and several 'road ragers' threw us the bird. Some felt sorry for us while others marveled at our journey. Some days our butts hurt. At other times, we rode like the wind. We became 'one' with nature.

We gobbled food like jet engines swallowing air. At night, noodle soup tasted like a seven course dinner at the Ritz, while rice and beans warmed out beings. We nibbled on apples, oranges, plums, nectarines, peaches, bananas and watermelon. The all-you-can-eat Pizza Hut and Golden Corral nearly killed us.

Everyone showed us kindness. This indeed, is a country made up of good, decent people. We witnessed the marvels of Yellowstone like Lewis and Clark and the mountain men saw it 200 years ago.

We traveled days without showers and stunk to high heaven. A shower became a thing of beauty and exhilaration.

We pedaled British Columbia, Montana, Wyoming, Colorado, Utah and New Mexico. We touched Mexico.

On a bicycle there is a sensory enhancement of the physical, that raises the spiritual aspect to new levels in the mind. We became kids again, but with a knowledge of our actions. People asked us why we toured on bicycles, but it was like trying to explain to a turtle what it was like to be a bird in flight. They couldn't know until they experienced it.

For those of us who pedal two wheels, it is enough to lift us into the journey and fly us through the moment into the next.

For Denis and me, it was an excellent adventure to end the century. We're looking forward to the next 100 years!

THE END

Epilogue

How is John Brown doing? John survived 10 sessions of chemotherapy. He endured 20 radiation therapies. He lost weight, got sick as a dog, battled against all odds, fought his way out of the chemo, got on a strict nutrition program, kept a positive mental attitude, got lots of love from his family and friends, and today, he is looking at a 100 percent recovery rate as of his last doctor evaluation. He's out riding his bike and sea kayaking each week. He is a powerful man with Iron Man determination. He's completed three Iron Man Triathlons. He's also a gentle man with a delicate spirit. With the qualities of his mind and spirit, he conquered cancer and won his life. In 2002, Denis, John and I met in Vancouver, Canada. We bicycled half way across Canada. At Banff, we turned south and pedaled down the Continental Divide. It was a most excellent adventure.

ABOUT THE AUTHOR

Living in Colorado, Frosty Wooldridge is an environmentalist, mountain climber, triathlete, dancer, Scuba diver, skier, writer and photographer. His features articles have appeared in national and international magazines including: BICYCLING, ADVENTURE CYCLIST and FREEWHEELING. He is the author of "HANDBOOK FOR TOURING BICYCLISTS"; "STRIKE THREE! TAKE YOUR BASE"; "AN EXTREME ENCOUNTER: ANTARCTICA"; "MOTORCYCLE ADVENTURE TO ALASKA"; "BICYCLING AROUND THE WORLD"; "BICYCLING THE CONTINENTAL DIVIDE" ; "RAFTING THE ROLLING THUNDER" ; "ARCTIC CIRCLE, NORWAY TO ATHENS, GREECE: BICYCLE ADVENTURE WITHOUT LIMITS" ; "THE NEXT ADDED 100 MILLION AMERICANS" Website: www.frostywooldridge.com

CPSIA information can be obtained at www.ICGtesting.com
Printed in the USA
BVOW04s0347120314

347358BV00001B/4/A